Digesting Foods and

Digesting Foods and Fads

Judi Nath

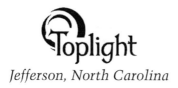

Jefferson, North Carolina

LIBRARY OF CONGRESS CATALOGUING-IN-PUBLICATION DATA

Names: Nath, Judi Lindsley, author.
Title: Digesting foods and fads / Judi Nath.
Description: Jefferson, North Carolina : Toplight, 2021 |
Includes bibliographical references and index.
Identifiers: LCCN 2021036184 | ISBN 9781476686400
(paperback : acid free paper) ∞
ISBN 9781476643991 (ebook)
Subjects: LCSH: Nutrition. | Diet. | BISAC: HEALTH & FITNESS /
Diet & Nutrition / General
Classification: LCC RA784 .N378 2021 | DDC 613.2—dc23
LC record available at https://lccn.loc.gov/2021036184

BRITISH LIBRARY CATALOGUING DATA ARE AVAILABLE

ISBN (print) 978–1–4766–8640–0
ISBN (ebook) 978–1–4766–4399–1

Front cover image © 2021 Lightspring/Shutterstock

Printed in the United States of America

Toplight is an imprint of McFarland & Company, Inc., Publishers

*Box 611, Jefferson, North Carolina 28640
www.toplightbooks.com*

Acknowledgments

My heartfelt gratitude to Bill Ober, MD, whose illustrations are simply unparalleled. There are no words to express my appreciation for your work in making this book better. In fact, the figures are so good that sometimes I wonder if words are even necessary. That is your treasured gift—and I'm fortunate to know you. Thank you to Claire Ober, RN, for your keen eye and deep interest in this product. Looking forward to many more years of friendship, dogs, beach walks, and conversation. Profound gratitude to Marianne Baker, MAT, who volunteered over pizza and beer to review pages. The conversations and laughs took us back to study abroad days and took us forward to life as we know it now. To my dear friends and colleagues, Anjali Dogra Gray, Ph.D., and Susan Shelangoskie, Ph.D., who read this book when it was just a chapter and a dream; thanks for encouraging me to expand on the idea. Paul, Lily, and Ethan Krieger were huge supports over many years. Their encouragement from up north kept me going many days! Martha Wolfe gets a round of applause for being such a great friend, timeless confidante, and excellent sign maker. Derek Perrigo, my biggest cheerleader and body-building inspiration, made me smile every day. He so believed this book needed an audience and was always ready with a marketing plan and cartwheel. As always, family, friends, colleagues, students, and peripheral supporters offered something every day, even when they didn't realize it. A great big hug to my husband, Mike, for his unwavering support through years of half-started chapters, partially-completed manuscripts, and middle-of-the-night ideas. To McFarland, a round of thanks for bringing this book to the world.

Table of Contents

Preface

We need it to survive, yet it can kill us. It can initiate a quite pleasurable experience or a gut-wrenching incident. It makes us who we are, however, it is not the essence of our being. We interact with it on a daily basis, and it is the foundation of a multibillion-dollar industry. What is *it*? *It* is food. And *it* is the subject of this book, *Digesting Foods and Fads*.

Digesting Foods and Fads is a curated source of nutrition information using the most current scientific evidence about the food we eat, how we should eat it, and where it comes from. It provides useful, honest information to avoid scams and swindlers, and we'll work through what foods you need and how your body uses the nutrients found in those necessary foods. There are no gimmicks.

More than 245 million people in the United States use the Internet, which means that 245 million people are exposed to lots of misinformation and scammers trying to make money. For example, despite filters and various blocks on my email accounts, I still receive hundreds of junk emails each day, most offering me quick fixes for health issues. Consider these subject lines related to diet and exercise that arrived within the past two hours:

- The Miracle Cure Big Pharma Doesn't Want You to Know About—Liquid Gold
- 50 lbs. in 61 Days: New No-Exercise "Skinny Pill" Melts Belly Fat—Show Off Your Body Again
- Newest Diet Product Has Unbelievable Results— The Real Shark Tank Keto!
- Real Weight Loss Results—Faster, Easier, and Cheaper— The Keto Diet

- 35+ Woman? You Deserve to Lose 47 Pounds NOW—BioHarmony
- New Skinny Pill Kills Too Much Fat? This Diet Is Sweeping the Nation—Forget Diet, and Exercise

If you were to fall victim to the clickbait, you'd find a lot of plausible sounding text. Text that seems easy to understand with just enough scientific terms to convince you the content is accurate. In most cases, it is nonsense, but you might not realize that until you've already given the scammers your credit card number.

Diet fads, nutritional supplements, and agricultural enterprises are multibillion-dollar industries that target our desire to be healthy. However, much of what's out there is nothing more than quackery and pseudoscience, couched within a smattering of facts. Food and food sources are inextricably linked to our lives because food is quite literally connected to living and life on this planet. This book will help you navigate the maze of fraud as it relates to eating well throughout our lives.

We want to lead healthy lives, and one factor in doing that involves understanding our options. To understand our options, we need health literacy, defined by the U.S. Department of Health and Human Services (HHS) as "the degree to which individuals have the capacity to obtain, process, and understand basic health information needed to make appropriate health decisions." As I write, only 12 percent of the American population has achieved health literacy. We can do better, and this book will help.

While the biochemistry of nutrients is complex, knowing what we should eat is not. Together, we'll walk through topics germane to our own bodies that do change across the lifespan, as well as those subjects relevant to us as human beings living within webs of societies, who are also tasked with being stewards of the Earth. Early topics lay the foundation for understanding how our bodies use nutrients and why those nutrients are important. These groundwork subjects include an overview of the digestive system and health, controlling weight and calories, and understanding the roles of carbohydrates, lipids (fats), proteins, vitamins, and minerals. Later topics deal with the functions of water, sustainable farming and eating practices, and ways to protect our environment through our food choices.

Along the way, we'll explore popular diets and food fads, while sprinkling in historical details (do you know why margarine was once colored pink?) and fun facts (backyard hens can lay up to 250 eggs per year!). The goal is to equip you with lifelong knowledge to make solid (and liquid) food choices for eating well, being an informed consumer, and knowing when something is bogus.

> "*You can fool all the people all the time if the advertising is right and the budget is big enough.*"—Joseph E. Levine (1905–1987); American producer, film distributor

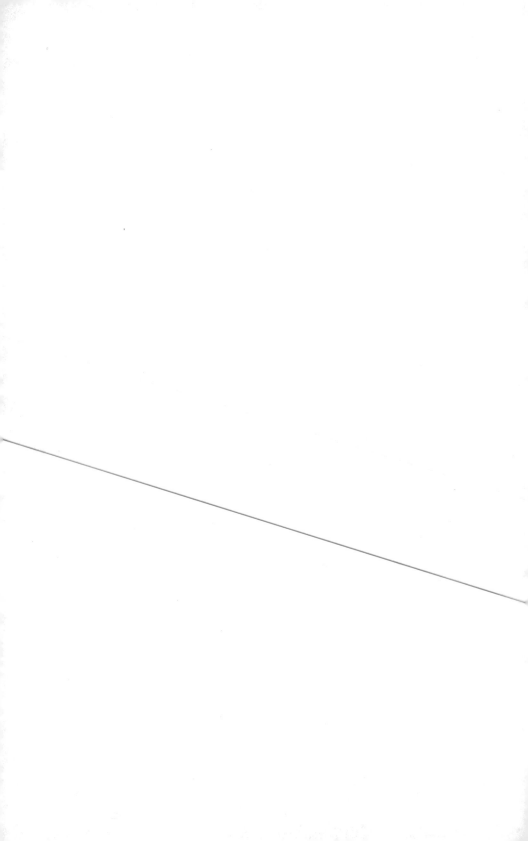

1

Animal, Vegetable or Mineral

Food and Health

Diet and Nutrition Confusion

Are you currently on some "diet"? If not, have you ever been on some "diet"? According to recent figures, Americans spend over $60 billion (that's with a "b") per year trying to lose weight. To give you some perspective, if you started counting now, and it took one second to count each number, it would take you 31 years, 251 days, seven hours, 46 minutes, and 39 seconds just to count to *one* billion. Now, multiply that by 60, that's more than 1,900 *years*! The point is that we spend a lot of money every year on self-help diet books, diet foods, diet fads, diet supplements, dieting, and gym memberships. The reality is that we *waste* a lot of money on these items.

Data show that the American population is consuming more calories and growing more obese, and as a consequence, the rates of diabetes, high blood pressure (hypertension), and heart disease are increasing. Various food factions claim to know what's best. Vegetarians continue to speak out against animal fat and point to the longevity seen among Asian peasants. Born-again meat-eaters blame white bread and grains and insist on eating all-meat diets that they claim will burn up their fat. The new entry on the diet front appears to be the gluten-free hipsters. In general, the public is baffled about what to do, so they follow TV ads, YouTube videos, and Internet gurus and consume whatever is advertised or expedient. Couple this with those fast food snacks that are readily available and bountiful. COVID-19 stay-at-home orders helped us reconnect with our pantries. Visit a hardware store to pick up a screwdriver and you discover you can buy potato chips at the checkout. Go to a clothing store and grab a chocolate bar on the way out. Quick and easy junk food is quite convenient. Nutrient-dense snacks are not.

Every time some family member, or friend, or kook on TV advocates for some new fad food or best diet known to humankind, I have found myself on the diet soapbox delivering a lecture to uninterested parties. After all, I wasn't touting a quick fix, or an easy pill to swallow, nor was I selling pre-packaged portions of the latest-greatest-scientifically-proven-to-shed-pounds-within-six-weeks powders. I thought I could convince these people—most of whom are quite intelligent—that what they were paying for was hooey. I had science to prove my point. As you probably have guessed, I lost nearly every time. So it was during a so-called important faculty meeting when I heard the high-paid speaker proclaim something stupid about dieting that I could take it no longer. I had been teaching nutrition science for years, so hearing hogwash was pretty hard to take. It was at that moment that I put pen to paper and began to write about diet and health for everyone, not just my students. I also like to think of it as showing the world that meetings actually can be productive!

If there is one area of science outside of astrophysics that is totally confusing, it has to be nutrition. One day this food is good for you. The next day it's bad for you. Eat this, don't eat that. Add the mountain of cookbooks for heart disease, diabetes, and disease prevention. Tack on the health gurus who have a plan for everything. Magnify the trends with thought-provoking documentaries. It's no wonder people are confused and often misinformed. This book is written to combat fads and misinformation by giving you solid science so you can make informed decisions about what goes into your mouth.

As a general rule, if some health craze is touted as the latest and greatest, suggests something along the lines of ingesting super foods daily, or tells you that a particular diet cures cancer, simply avoid it. Extremism—regardless of the field—is crazy. We are human beings with hundreds of thousands of years of evolution to deal with. Our physiology strives for homeostasis, the tendency toward a relatively stable balance. Such equilibrium is not based on extremes but rather on maintaining values within a range. For example, throughout the day, temperature fluctuates, blood sugar levels rise and fall, and sleepiness waxes and wanes. These variations are all normal. We are genetically programmed for variation and the "what ifs."

Let's delve in by looking at the term *diet*. The word *diet* comes to us via Latin from the Greek word *diaita*, meaning *a way of life*. Specifically, diet refers to the food you routinely eat, thus it is your personal, habitual eating habits. You should not "go on" a diet, but rather eat nutritious food. Sage advice for prime functioning and optimum health involves moderation, while maintaining a mixed diet rich in fruits, vegetables, nuts, and whole grains with limited processed foods. Along with healthy eating, keeping moving and exercising are keys to optimal well-being.

Our issues do not stem from lack of dieting, but from our diets themselves. First and foremost, we must consider human biology. Once we accept and understand the very basic scientific principles underlying our physiology, it'll be easier to accept that *diet* really means "the food we eat in accordance with our activity level necessary to achieve our desired weight." No pun intended, but that sentence was a mouthful. Our diet is what we eat and how much we eat. The truth is that on a daily basis, we require six major nutrients: carbohydrates, lipids (fats), proteins, vitamins, minerals, and water. That's it. Truly. It's that simple.

We hear a lot about nutrition, but what *is* nutrition? Nutrition is a term that seems to be synonymous with good food. However, from a biological perspective, nutrition is the food and water required by your body for normal, physiological functioning. That functioning includes generating energy, maintaining organ functions, growing, and enabling activity.

How much food and water we need depends on lots of factors. It's not a one-size-fits-all equation. Age, underlying medical conditions, environment, medications, pregnancy, breastfeeding, illness, activities, and other individualized factors have to be taken into account when determining food type and caloric intake.

Calories are energy packets found in food, and all the food we eat takes several paths within the body. Once inside the body, food is broken down into its component nutrients, used, stored, or excreted as waste. What the body does with the nutrients depends on immediate needs. If there is no immediate purpose, the nutrients are stored for later use or excreted. Actually, your body is the world's best recycler and has been recycling long before the whole "Green Movement"! Carbohydrates, fats, and proteins—the macronutrients—are broken down to provide energy, while vitamins and minerals—the micronutrients—aid the macronutrients. Water is a macronutrient, but it does not provide energy; it helps with chemical processing of nutrients.

Despite the fact that there are only six major nutrients, diets and diet fads have been highly commercialized. Why are there so many diets, diet fads, diet supplements, and advertisements devoted to our food? Money is one reason and weight loss focus is another. Besides companies being able to make large sums of cash peddling diets, many people really do want to lose weight. This is especially ironic considering that the World Hunger and Poverty Facts and Statistics showed that millions of people in *developed* countries—that includes the United States—are malnourished. A systematic study conducted across 195 countries showed that poor diet—consuming low amounts of healthy foods such as whole grains and fruits and high amounts of sodium, accounts for one in five deaths globally.

Malnutrition is faulty nutrition that results from malabsorption, poor diet, or overeating. Malabsorption occurs with some medical conditions in which nutrients cannot be absorbed. In such cases, a person may be eating enough, but their bodies cannot extract and absorb the nutrients. For example, if the pancreas isn't working properly, a person may not be able to digest and absorb carbohydrates.

Poor diets are responsible for more deaths than tobacco and high blood pressure. Poor diets can lead to malnutrition because the food that is eaten doesn't contain the right amount of nutrients. Diets consisting of single foods or just a few types of food may contain enough calories, but not the necessary nutrients. So a person could eat only apples and whole grain rice—which are good, nutritious foods—but if that is all they are eating, they won't be consuming all the necessary nutrients.

Then there is malnourishment that also occurs with overeating, which is a case of enough food, but the food is energy dense and deficient in nutrients. Diets high in junk foods, which contain lots of calories but very few nutrients are examples of overeating with little nutritional value. These are called *empty calories*. For example, if you ate nothing but pretzels, potato chips, and ice cream, you'd have plenty of calories, but these calories lack the necessary nutrients.

Malnourishment is particularly disturbing because being underweight is just as dangerous as being overweight. Anorexia nervosa and cancer cachexia are two different conditions of malnourishment accompanied by profound weight loss. Both look alike, can lead to a person being severely malnourished, and can both cause death, but their underlying causes and underlying mechanisms are different.

Throughout these pages, you'll get the sense of what constitutes good scientific support for best eating practices and well-being. The major formula for a good, longer, healthier life has generally been to eat right and get plenty of exercise. It all sounds very simple, but questions arise: What are we supposed to eat? How much and what kind of exercise are we supposed to get? How do you get started on this, even if you want to change an unhealthy habit? Or how do you make healthy living even better? Science is giving us clues about what the body truly needs, and there is some sorting out of the many options. However, just watching your diet and the bathroom scales is not enough. We have to be willing to move, if only to walk a half-hour a day briskly.

Think of these pages as a nutrition primer of sorts. A guide to understanding nutritional needs, helping you maintain desirable weight for a lifetime, and providing information so you can avoid wasting money on sham diets. If you get no further than these paragraphs, know that some nutrition concepts have withstood the test of time, various nutrition controversies will likely persist, and all the answers are not known. However, using evidence-based science is always the best choice when making decisions regarding health and wellness. Read and digest (pun intended)!

Nutrition Science, Nutritional Experts and Reputable Sources

The foundation for this book, nutrition science, is a relative newcomer as an academic discipline. Chemistry, biology, biochemistry, medicine, physics, anthropology, and sociology—among other areas—had to be invented first before nutrition science could emerge as a scientific study. In fact, nutrition science dates back to around the 18th century, and clinical nutrition as an academic field is an even newer arrival, originating around the 20th century. For perspective, chemistry has been around since 1000 BCE, medicine since the fifth century, and physics has origins in the fourth century.

Think of clinical nutrition as applied nutrition. As a science, clinical nutrition is the specialty that views the interaction between nutrition and health and the role nutrition plays in treating disease. For example, until the end of the 18th century, scurvy affected poorly nourished sailors. As a disease, scurvy caused swollen gums and poor wound healing. Its cause is vitamin C deficiency so the treatment is a relatively easy fix: eat foods like oranges and other citrus fruits that contain vitamin C.

By definition, nutrition science is the branch of study that examines how the body uses carbohydrates, fats, proteins, vitamins, minerals, and water. People are often frustrated—and rightly so—with nutrition news because it seems as though some food that was good for you yesterday, should be avoided today. You're familiar with such news: Coffee is bad, coffee is good! Eggs are bad, eggs are good! The reasons for such disparity are the direct result of the "newness" of the nutrition science discipline itself, coupled with the fact that studying nutritional effects on living, breathing humans is hard to do. Genes, lifestyle, environment, and other not-yet-known factors come into play. Plus, we humans are not all alike. Because we humans are not all alike, it's also extremely difficult to study nutrition in people without confining them in the same environment, exposing them to the same activities, and feeding them the same food for a prolonged time. Obviously, this is not something people or researchers are eager to do.

As we progress through these pages, we'll focus on the role nutrients play in health and disease. But first, we need to know reliable sources of food information. This is tough, because few people are actually licensed to dispense such information and the supplement industry is largely unregulated. But we have to begin somewhere. Think about where you, personally, receive your nutrition information. Does it come from advertising? Your physician? Television? The Internet? The nutrition label on food packaging? In the United States, registered dietitians and licensed dietitians are qualified to dispense nutrition information. Yet, even these terms are confusing because it's hard to differentiate between "registered" and "licensed" as they seem like synonyms. Whether "registered" or "licensed" is used depends on the state in which you live. Registered and licensed dietitians have undergraduate and/or advanced degrees in nutrition and have passed examinations qualifying them in their field. Thus, either are reliable sources of nutrition information.

Another professional who also dispenses nutrition information is a "nutritionist." Although it sounds as though dietitian and nutritionist are interchangeable terms, these professions are related, but they are not the same. The two are differentiated by their legal restrictions. Whereas dietitians pass licensing exams to become registered or licensed and must adhere to government regulations, this does not always apply to nutritionists. While some states do require nutritionists to have an occupational license to practice, other states require nothing. This means that you could be getting advice from a nutritionist who has no education, training, or work experience in the field and is armed with little more than an Internet certificate—if that. You could also be getting very sound nutritional advice from somebody who has studied nutrition and has a degree in nutrition, but who is not licensed. Still confused? Probably, because this is still a little crazy. Plus, dietitian can also be spelled dietician.

Then, there is this from the *Consumer Health Digest* #20–30 which summarized an article by Marton, Wang, Barabási, and Ioannidis thusly: A team of researchers has analyzed the top 100 bestselling nutrition-focused books during the period 2008 to 2015 based on Google Books summaries, online information about the authors, and text analysis of seven of the top ten books available in electronic form. They found the following:

- Eighty of the summaries mentioned weight loss or weight management.
- Of the summaries that specified a weight, the stated program lengths and numbers of pounds that could be lost varied greatly with medians of 21 days and 15.5 pounds.
- 31 of the summaries referred to claims that following the nutrition advice provided could cure or prevent diseases.
- Specific diseases claimed to be curable or preventable by following the nutrition advice included diabetes (in 15 book summaries), heart disease (in 12), cancer (11), dementia (8), arthritis (6), autoimmune disorders (5), Parkinson's disease (3), autism spectrum disorder (3), and depression (3). Following the nutrition advice provided was claimed in 13 book summaries to increase energy levels and in 7 to increase lifespan.
- The 100 summaries showed very little consistency in terms of what were the key components of a beneficial diet.
- Of the 83 unique authors, 33.7 percent had a medical degree and 6.0 percent had a Ph.D. degree, while about half of the authors had no graduate degree.

The paper includes a sample list taken from the summaries of 16 nutritional claims that the researchers consider disputable and/or unsubstantiated. The researchers wrote:

> In all, our assessment of the summaries of best-selling books on nutrition shows that they may provide information or misinformation about very important matters and they are a heterogeneous mix. We cannot exclude that some of them may be providing sound or even excellent advice, but it is likely that many, probably the large majority, contain substantial misinformation and claims that have no scientific foundation.

Here's another curious tidbit to add to the mix: Physicians may be primary sources of nutrition information, yet according to a survey of the status of nutrition education in medical schools, only 27 percent of U.S. medical schools met the minimum 25 required hours of nutrition education set by the National Academy of Sciences. According to David Eisenberg, adjunct associate professor of nutrition at the Harvard T.H. Chan School of Public Health, only about one-fifth of American medical schools require students to take a nutrition course. That's not to say that physicians are not reliable sources for nutrition education. They and plenty of other people can be good sources of information. And, by the end of this book, you should have all the information you need as well. Since we all need food and water to survive, a college degree in basic life functions is not necessary. What helps us though, is a solid foundation about nutrients and how our body uses them. And knowing where to find valid, reliable nutrition information for those times we don't know also helps us make wise decisions.

Where are we getting our nutrition information? A quick Google Internet search of the term "nutrition" resulted in nearly 1.3 trillion sites! Obviously, we get our nutrition information from a variety of sources, but the Internet and its sites are probably high on the list. This is why we need to recognize reputable sites, read carefully, and have a solid understanding of very basic nutrition science.

Media oftentimes sensationalize findings to grab our attention. Yet, scientists are in the trenches looking for trends, researching claims, and evaluating the data. Four government agencies with reputable scientists who are involved in research, nutrition monitoring, and public policy in the United States are the (1) Department of Health and Human Services (DHHS), (2) U.S. Food and Drug Administration (FDA), (3) U.S. Department of Agriculture (USDA), and (4) Centers for Disease Control and Prevention (CDC). Other reliable sources are listed at the end of this book in the Bibliography under Reputable General Websites.

Nutrients

Why do we eat? Aside from the fact that food tastes good and eating is a social experience, we eat to obtain energy. It's a tad bit more complicated, though, because it's not enough just to eat. We could eat three pounds of bacon and two bags of potato chips and have plenty of *calories*, but we wouldn't have the appropriate *nutrients*. In fact, this is an example of how a person could be overweight but malnourished.

What we eat is as important as *how much* we eat. We've all heard that we need nutritious food, so let's begin with the nutrients that the body requires.

What are nutrients? A nutrient is a substance that provides essential components for cellular and bodily functions. Again, here is a list of the six major nutrients the body needs: carbohydrates, fats, proteins, vitamins, minerals, and water. The first three are the only nutrients that have calories. Think of calories as energy. Carbohydrates and proteins each contain four calories per gram, while fats contain nine calories per gram. You read that correctly: Fat provides more than double the calories of carbohydrates and proteins. Vitamins, minerals, and water have zero calories. Thus, the calorie count of food depends on the amounts of carbohydrates, fats, and proteins it contains. And when it comes to nutrients with calories, our bodies play favorites. Scientists call this "preferential nutrient use." Our innate biochemistry dictates what gets used and when: Carbohydrates are used first, followed by fats, followed by proteins.

Our diets, however, are as individualized as we are. Thus, it's a bit tricky to find the one-size-fits-all diet. To illustrate, consider that Olympic speed skater Apolo Ohno consumed anywhere between 2,500 to 8,000 calories a day, depending on his activity level. Olympic swimmer Michael Phelps consumed 12,000 calories a day while training. These guys also burned a boatload of calories. Sedentary folks would gain weight eating that many calories.

Nutrients follow complex biochemical pathways from the moment we eat them until the moment we excrete them. Carbohydrates, fats, and proteins have separate metabolic pathways that are specific for each nutrient. However, they do intersect depending on a person's nutrient status. The point is that the metabolism of each nutrient is complicated, which is why many people can be tricked by schmoozy advertising. It's a classic case of a person not knowing what they don't know. But that's okay because we're learning here.

Two basic biochemical pathways occur in the body: anabolic pathways for building up and catabolic pathways for breaking down. Anabolic pathways—or anabolism—make complex molecules from simpler ones. For example, anabolism is a constructive pathway because it takes components of carbohydrates, fats, and proteins to form tissues and store energy. Catabolic pathways—or catabolism—break down complex molecules into simpler ones. For example, complex molecules are broken down to produce energy and waste. Together, anabolism and catabolism make up our metabolism. Foods and drinks provide the necessary calories to make these processes happen because both anabolism and catabolism require energy. You've heard of metabolism, quite likely in terms of somebody having a fast metabolism or slow one.

The amount of energy ingested is measured in calories, and the average person needs about 1,500 to 2,000 calories per day. Of course, there are no average individuals, so these calories vary depending on physical activity, body size, age, height, and health status. The nutrition type also affects our body's metabolic rate. For example, carbohydrates require less energy to process than do proteins. One thing is certain, if you accumulate an extra 3,500 calories, that will add one pound of body weight.

Recall that calories are associated with only carbohydrates, fats, and proteins. Vitamins, minerals, and water do not have any calories. That said, you've likely heard a person comment, "Since I started taking vitamins, I have more energy!" This is a false statement because vitamins have no calories and without calories you can't have more energy. It could be a psychological benefit, or, if a person were deficient in a particular vitamin, they might feel better.

If you wanted to lose weight, consuming only water, vitamins, and minerals is a sure way to do so. However, you cannot live on just these three nutrients. In order to survive, you still need all six types of nutrients in combination because each has a particular role in biochemical pathways. These biochemical pathways ensure an energy source to fuel and repair our cells and enable cellular function. Succinctly, our cells need all six to function correctly.

To understand much about what we eat and why we eat it, we need to look at marketing against the backdrop of evolution. For years, we have been shaped by marketing and advertisements. We've been told that in order to build muscle, we need to eat animal protein. While protein is essential to building muscle, we don't need to get that protein from animals. There are other sources of perfectly good protein. If we step back and think about this logically, does it make sense that the very animals we eat for our protein source are themselves vegetarians? In the natural world, cows eat plants; hence, they are herbivores. Their teeth and digestive systems are specialized for consuming plants, deriving nutrients from plant-based diets, and building the very muscles we consume. We humans began our evolutionary journey as herbivores. Indeed, most primates are herbivores and even today, apes survive on a plant-based diet. We'll look at each of these nutrients and how the body uses them in the upcoming chapters. Before we get there, we need to look at the role of governmental policy in shaping what we eat. That begins with the U.S. Dietary Guidelines. The government of Canada also establishes a similar food guide.

U.S. Dietary Guidelines for Americans

Every five years, the United States Department of Agriculture (USDA) works with the U.S. Department of Health and Human Services to publish the Dietary Guidelines for Americans. However, the group ultimately in charge of creating the guidelines is the Dietary Guidelines Advisory Committee. These guidelines exist to help people make sound dietary nutritional choices and to give healthcare providers recommendations for healthy eating.

We haven't always had such guidelines. Before we had the Dietary Guidelines for Americans, American chemist Wilbur Olin Atwater (May 3, 1844–September 22, 1907) was at work studying human nutrition and metabolism. He ultimately developed the Atwater System, a methodology for calculating the energy found in food. In 1894, he published dietary recommendations for Americans, which were the precursor to what we have today. As a scientist, he was studying how the digestive system functions and how various nutrients are broken down by the body. He was laying the foundation for nutrition science, and what he said in 1894 still rings true: "We live not upon what we eat, but upon what we digest."

Modeling the Atwater System, the first modern-day guidelines were published in 1980. Several iterations pre-date what we have today. More recent visual representations of the guidelines were the Food Guide Pyramid followed by the MyPyramid, which is now replaced by MyPlate. There is great importance to these guidelines because they serve as the general nutritional playbook for clinicians, dieticians, scientists, and policy makers. To provide a contextual framework, here's a brief history of our present-day guidelines.

From 1916 to the 1930s, the USDA's guides "Food for Young Children" and "How to Select Food" established guidance based on food groups and household measures. Its focus was on "protective foods," which we needed to maintain adequate nutrition. The 1940s version, "A Guide to Good Eating (Basic Seven)," was complex and included the number of servings needed from each of seven food groups per day. Those seven food groups were (1) green and yellow vegetables; (2)

oranges, tomatoes, grapefruit; (3) potatoes and other vegetables and fruits; (4) milk and milk products; (5) meat, poultry, fish, or eggs; (6) bread, flour, and cereals; and (7) butter and fortified margarine.

By the 1950s, dietary guidelines added fitness to the mix. From 1956 to the 1970s, Food for Fitness, A Daily Food Guide (Basic Four), provided goals for nutrient adequacy from four food groups. Remember those four basic food groups? They were milk, meat, fruits and vegetables, and breads and cereals. Within each group were representative examples. The year 1979 brought us the Hassle-Free Daily Food Guide. This one was based on the basic four but added a fifth group that highlighted moderate intake of fats, sweets, and alcohol. Then, in 1984 we had the Food Wheel: A Pattern for Daily Food Choices. It was a total diet approach that also provided daily amounts of food within each of the five categories from the previous guidelines. The Food Wheel formed the basis for the 1992 Food Guide Pyramid. The Food Guide Pyramid was a little more sophisticated because it was developed using consumer research; focused on variety, moderation, and proportion; and used a total diet approach that gave goals for nutrition adequacy and moderation. Foods forming the base of the pyramid were the ones to be eaten in the greatest amounts. As one moved toward the peak, food servings diminished. Bread, cereal, rice and pasta formed the base at six to 11 daily servings. Sharing the next level were the vegetable group with three to five servings and the fruit group with two to four servings. Nearing the top was the milk, yogurt, and cheese group with two to three servings and the meat, poultry, fish, dry beans, eggs and nuts group with two to three servings. At the tip top were fats, oils and sweets, which were to be consumed sparingly. The visual representations of each of the guidelines helped tremendously in understanding food types and proportions.

We're getting close to the current guidelines. In 2005, we had the MyPyramid Food Guidance System. This one looked very much like the former pyramid, but with the added band for oils and the addition of physical activity. There was also an accompanying website: www.MyPyramid.gov. In 2011, the "My" theme continued, and the pyramid was retooled into MyPlate. Categories were pie-shaped icons within a dinner plate circle. If you are familiar with the board game *Trivial Pursuit*, envision each category as a pie piece placed in the circular token. The words (1) fruits, (2) grains, (3) vegetables, (4) protein, and (5) dairy (on the side) were used in place of food pictures. One had to be literate in English to understand it.

Today, we have ChooseMyPlate. Its five categories are (1) fruits, (2) vegetables, (3) grains, (4) dairy, and (5) protein foods. People are left wondering how something so germane to life, i.e., eating food to survive, can be so complicated. It's really not extraordinarily complicated. The beauty of science is that when we learn more about something, we adapt. The bane of government is that it is greatly influenced by money. And these guidelines are not exempt from financial influence.

Why would guidelines be influenced by non-scientific interests? Because industry has much to gain if their products can make it on the guidelines. Moreover, these guidelines influence many government programs including the National School Lunch Program, School Breakfast Program, Special Supplemental Nutrition Program for Women, Infants, and Children (WIC), the U.S. Department of Health and Human Services Administration on Aging, the Older Americans Act Nutrition Service programs, the Department of Defense's meal rations for military personnel, and the Department of Veterans Affairs for the VA Hospital System.

As you can see, many agencies depend on the nutritional guidelines. Thus, its implications are widespread. Some of the biggest lobbyists in Washington, D.C., are in the meat and dairy industries, which is why you'll also see both red meat and dairy products listed on the guidelines—this despite the fact that humans need neither. The guidelines are not all bad, though. They state that we should get plenty of fruits, vegetables, and whole grains; protein should come from a variety of sources; dairy should be fat-free or low-fat; sodium, trans-fats, and saturated fats should be limited; and no more than 10 percent of the total calories consumed daily should be from added sugars. Yet, critics feel the guidelines don't go far enough. Current dietary guidelines recommend that you eat:

- 45 percent–65 percent of your daily calories from carbohydrates,
- 20 percent–35 percent from fat, and
- 10 percent–35 percent from protein.

Each time there is a revision, there is also controversy. Every time. Many reasons cited are legitimate. Nutrition scientists state that the convened panels fail to look through the most rigorous scientific studies to arrive at their conclusions, confirmation bias looms large, there are oftentimes non-disclosed conflicts of interest, and food lobbyists influence what does and doesn't get placed on the guidelines. But you can't list everything, which is why you need a solid foundation in the basics.

You simply need to know enough to make sound choices and to know when something is bunk. And that's why you need to know how twisting scientific facts can advance monetary missions. We see it in diet fads. We see it in marketing. And we see it when businesses want to confuse the general public. Don't be fooled.

Have you heard of Exponent, Inc.? It was formerly known as The Failure Group, Inc. It is a company that claims to be a multi-disciplinary engineering and scientific consulting firm that solves engineering, scientific, regulatory, and business issues facing their clients. If you go to their website, they look and sound like a legitimate organization whose mission is to advance scientific principles. In actuality, their mission is to dupe the public. Any time a company needs a "hired gun," they call on Exponent, Inc. to get them out of their legal wrangling. Exponent, Inc. is basically a science-for-hire company that will twist facts, use bias reporting, and frame it within a scientific context to make their case. They've been used by ExxonMobil in their case in which they lied about the risks of burning fossil fuels. They were used by the tobacco industry in their false claims about the hazards of tobacco. They were used by the National Football League (NFL) in the Deflategate scandal. The food industry is now using Exponent, Inc. to undermine public health policies by manipulating data.

Tactics used by hired guns of the food industry are aimed at casting doubt on solid science. In fact, internal memos show that doubt *is* the product. Casting doubt is the best means of competing with facts that exist within the minds of the general public. It is manipulation pure and simple. If you see advertisements contradicting scientific evidence, be skeptical.

Food Labels

Whenever you look at a nutrition label on food—called nutrition facts—you'll notice that food components are listed as amount per serving in grams (g), milligrams (mg), and percent of daily value. An ingredient list will also be on the package label. Most labels make your eyes go bonkers. The FDA even has a website to help you understand and use the nutrition facts label. Each label is standardized to include an overview of nutrition facts and lists serving size, calories (and calories from fat), nutrients (and those that should be limited), other nutrients that you should get enough of, footnotes citing percent daily values, and a quick guide to percent daily value (% DV).

If you're health conscious, a good rule of thumb is to eat foods with the fewest ingredients. Raw fruits, raw vegetables, and whole foods typically fall into this category. The ingredient list identifies food components in descending order, listing the substance that is in the greatest amount first with the last item being the one with the least amount. In the case of a bag of potato chips, a common staple in the American diet, the first ingredient will likely be potatoes, followed by vegetable oil, rounded out by salt. Then, you'll see "Nutrition Facts." This lists the serving size, calories, and the percentage of nutrients. For our potato chip example, about 15 chips make up a serving (around one ounce) and that serving contains 160 calories. Listed under the Nutrition Facts you'll also see total fat (saturated and trans), cholesterol, sodium, potassium, total carbohydrate (dietary fiber and total sugars), protein, and various vitamins and minerals. We'll look at the various nutrients later in the chapter and throughout this book. But the Nutrition Facts label identifies the amount of nutrients by weight and percentage of daily value for daily diets of 2,000 calories.

At the beginning of 2020, new nutrition facts labels went into effect. The purpose of the new label is to reflect how we actually eat, so you'll see side-by-side comparisons for a single serving and for the entire package. Figure 1.1 shows the new dual column food label identifying nutrition facts per serving and per container.

Recall the dietary guidelines previously discussed as you review this food label. Keep in mind that these are ranges so they vary depending on many factors. Going back

Nutrition Facts

2 servings per container
Serving size 1 cup (255g)

	Per serving		Per container	
Calories	**220**		**440**	
		% DV*		% DV*
Total Fat	5g	6%	10g	13%
Saturated Fat	2g	10%	4g	20%
Trans Fat	0g		0g	
Cholesterol	15mg	5%	30mg	10%
Sodium	240mg	10%	480mg	21%
Total Carb.	35g	13%	70g	25%
Dietary Fiber	6g	21%	12g	43%
Total Sugars	7g		14g	
Incl. Added Sugars	4g	8%	8g	16%
Protein	9g		18g	
Vitamin D	5mcg	25%	10mcg	50%
Calcium	200mg	15%	400mg	30%
Iron	1mg	6%	2mg	10%
Potassium	470mg	10%	940mg	20%

* The % Daily Value (DV) tells you how much a nutrient in a serving of food contributes to a daily diet. 2,000 calories a day is used for general nutrition advice.

Figure 1.1 New dual column nutrition labels show nutrition facts per serving and per container (from FDA).

to our potato chip bag, those 15 chips contain 5 percent of your total carbohydrate for the day, 16 percent of fat, and 0 percent of protein. Since potato chips are devoid of protein, you would suffer from protein energy malnutrition if all you ate were chips. You'd also have other vitamin and mineral deficiencies as well.

Food Justice

Before we talk about actual food, it is important to discuss food justice. Why do we have so much wealth and yet we have poverty? How can we have food surplus and yet people live in food deserts? Living in the United States is a bit of a paradox. We have lots of resources, and smart people, and plenty of food, yet accessing food can be a challenge. Accessing quality, fresh food can be a greater challenge. Add to that food costs. Even if the food is there, it may not be accessible. Studies have shown that African Americans, Native Americans, and Latinx people are less likely to live in areas with access to fresh, healthy food. That is, the stores aren't there, creating so-called food deserts. This has genuine health consequence because these communities also experience higher rates of diabetes than other communities. As I write, we're in the midst of a pandemic and the facts are astounding: COVID-19 infected people with diabetes have worse outcomes than those without diabetes.

Other studies have also shown that if you look at this scenario through the lens of income, even if the food were available, many people of color simply can't afford it or don't have the time to shop for healthy food and/or cook from scratch. If you're scratching your head pondering this, think about working two jobs to support your family. If you did have time to shop, would you also have time to cook a well-balanced meal? There are only so many hours in a day.

The pandemic has also taught us about the food chain as one-eighth of the U.S. labor force is linked to the food system. Additionally, food workers themselves are treated less than fair and have a disproportionate number of workers affected with COVID-19. Although definitions vary by state, departments of health generally define a food worker as anyone who works with unpackaged food, food equipment, or utensils; is responsible for food storage, preparation, or display; or who works with any surface where people place unwrapped food. Many states require food workers to have a valid food worker card. Food workers are also more likely to be underpaid and lack health insurance all while working in unsafe environments rampant with workforce exploitation.

When we look at farm ownership, people of color are also under-represented. This is deeply rooted in our history of racism and land theft from Native peoples. Meatpacking jobs, listed as one of the most dangerous jobs in America, is an industry in which one-third of the workforce are immigrants and undocumented workers. Meat processing plants tend to be unsanitary places where workers have very low wages and amputations are common.

Food justice also encompasses caring for our citizenry. A branch of the USDA is Food and Nutrition Service (FNS). The goal of FNS is to end hunger and obesity through the administration of 15 federal nutrition assistance programs, including Supplemental Nutrition Assistance Program (SNAP), Special Supplemental Nutrition Program for Women, Infants, and Children (WIC), and school meals. One in four Americans receives assistance from an FNS nutrition program each year.

Formerly known as food stamps, SNAP provides food assistance to about 11.8 percent of the United States population. In 2020 the Trump administration worked to tighten access to SNAP by various measures including making 18- to 49-year-olds who are able-bodied, childless, and without people to care for, work 20 hours per week to qualify. This would be waived if they lived in an area of high unemployment as newly defined by the administration. Via temporary flexibility provided by the Families First Coronavirus Act of March 2020, the cuts to SNAP participation did not happen—in fact, SNAP grew. In January 2020, participation was 37,100,836, but by May 2021 it became 42 million Americans. In addition, the mandatory work requirement was temporarily suspended, plus the USDA encouraged states to make access to SNAP enrollment easier. Families First also gave a temporary boost to emergency supplementary benefits and school meal replacement benefits. These have been strengthened and extended by the Biden Administration.

On the surface and as talking points by politicians across the spectrum, this might seem to be a reasonable plan. Digging deeper and looking through a broader scope, we know that it is a vital part of the food safety net for low-income Americans. The program is very effective in reducing hunger, food insecurity, and poverty—and by extension reducing the health effects brought upon by these variables. It is a complex issue and the program is protected from total disbandment because it is couched within the Farm Bill (Pub L 115–334). The Farm Bill is in place to protect agribusiness. In fact, SNAP and the Farm Bill are linked: Congress cannot vote to pass agribusiness without passing SNAP at the same time.

No doubt, SNAP is expensive to operate. The total cost in 2019 was

$60.6 billion dollars and it provided benefits to 40.3 million adults and children. This total is about one in eight Americans. Plus, administrative costs totaled $4.4 billion. People receiving SNAP benefits do not get cash. Instead, they receive benefits through Electronic Benefit Transfer (EBT) debit cards, via an arrangement between the USDA and banks.

What can people who use SNAP benefits purchase? They may buy food, beverages, food seeds, and food plants. They may not buy alcoholic beverages, tobacco products, pet food, dietary supplements, hot foods, or non-food items.

In reality, SNAP is about helping poor people and those living in poverty. This is oftentimes a tough issue because living in poverty is difficult to understand simply through reading about it. Living with it or through it provides a different perspective. It's interesting to note that attitudes toward the poor (as a group) and public assistance are rooted in English Poor Laws of the 1600s. Poor Laws authorized benefits for poor people, and they were funded through public taxes. These laws viewed poor people as unworthy and viewed poverty as a personal choice, not one of misfortune or an issue with the economic system. Charles Dickens wrote about these laws that prevented starvation, but simultaneously created poor houses, required people to work—and punished them for not working—and encouraged child labor.

While public welfare has a long history, it's important to remember public wellness, because that's really the purpose of welfare. If you look at its word roots, it means to fare well, implying the health, happiness, and fortune of a person. And that's why administrators see the benefit of public assistance programs and published research studies confirm that SNAP is beneficial. In 2017, SNAP lifted 3.4 million people out of poverty. Of that number, nearly half were children. These are children who cannot control the environments in which they are born or live.

WIC is another federally-funded program aimed at saving lives and improving the health of nutritionally at-risk women, infants, and children (WIC). The Food and Nutrition Service of the USDA oversees this special supplemental nutrition program. It has earned the reputation of being one of the most successful federally-funded nutrition programs in the United States. Numerous studies have confirmed WICs benefits, including improving birth outcomes and containing health care costs. It has improved diets, diet-related outcomes, infant feeding practices, immunization rates, cognitive development, and pre-conceptional nutritional status.

Who is eligible for WIC? Pregnant women (during pregnancy and up to six weeks after birth), postpartum women (up to six months after birth), breastfeeding women (up to infant's first birthday), infants (up to the infant's first birthday), and children (up to the child's fifth birthday). People using the service must have income at or below standards set by the state, which is between 100 percent of the federal poverty guidelines but not more than 185 percent of federal poverty income guidelines. In 2018, WIC cost the federal government $5.3 billion and served 6.87 million people. Of that 6.87 million, 3.52 were children and 1.71 were infants.

Best Ways to Prepare Food

Time to turn our attention to food preparation. To get the most out of the food we eat, it's good to know the best way to prepare it for optimal nutrition. Surprisingly, raw is not always better. Cooking vegetables can break down tough structures thereby enabling the body to absorb the nutrients better. When carrots and spinach are cooked before they are eaten, the result is higher blood levels of beta carotene, which is converted to vitamin A in the body. Beta carotene is a red-orange plant pigment found in yellow and orange fruits and vegetables. Examples of these are cantaloupes, mangoes, pumpkins, papayas, carrots, and sweet potatoes. Beta carotene is also found in green leafy vegetables such as spinach and kale, but the green pigment, chlorophyll, masks the color.

Mentioning sweet potatoes brings up another question that is frequently asked: What is the difference between sweet potatoes and yams? Both are tuber vegetables, but they belong to different plant families, have differing nutrition content, and taste differently. Sweet potatoes, known by their scientific name *Ipomoea batatas*, are edible, climbing plants with pinkish orange, slightly sweet flesh that originated in Central America. North Carolina is the largest producer of sweet potatoes in the United States, but its name is a misnomer as it is only distantly related to potatoes. Yams, known scientifically as *Dioscorea*—with many species—are also climbing plants grown largely in tropical and subtropical countries, with 95 percent grown in Africa. The flesh varies in color from white or yellow to purple or pink. Taste-wise, they are drier and starchier than sweet potatoes and not commonly found in U.S. supermarkets.

So, if they are not commonly found in the United States, why are the names commonly used interchangeably? The likely reason is that when African slaves first encountered sweet potatoes, it reminded them of the vegetable they knew, so they called sweet potatoes, "nyami," which translated into "yam" in English. There is also a "mythconception" that eating yams increases the chances of having twins in Nigerian women. One night while I was teaching nutrition and the reproductive system, one of my Nigerian students told me that in her village, many women had twins and they attributed the high rate to eating yams. A possible reason is that yams may contain phytoestrogens, which stimulate the release of multiple eggs in females, allowing for a greater chance of two eggs being fertilized. The influence of yams on twinning has not been borne out in the scientific literature; nonetheless, twinning is indeed common in Nigeria.

In addition to making more vitamins available, cooking can also help increase mineral availability. As a general rule, cooking time, temperature, and additional liquid should be kept to a minimum. Thus, steaming is oftentimes (not the case for carrots) better than boiling. However, you can recapture nutrients lost to the water after boiling vegetables by using the water in some other dish you are preparing. For example, water used to boil potatoes can be used for the gravy.

Microwaving is a good option. When foods are microwaved, they generally retain most of their nutrients. An exception is cauliflower, which loses many nutrients after boiling and microwaving. The next best method is sautéing, using a healthy oil like extra-virgin olive oil. Because many vitamins in vegetables are fat-soluble, the oil increases the absorption of the phytonutrients, the plant substances that are beneficial to human health. From here, griddling, baking, and roasting are next in order of the best methods of cooking to preserve nutrients.

Griddling involves using a heavy pan or a separate flat griddle with a little bit of oil. This is not grilling, which is done over charcoal, wood, or propane flame. In terms of baking and roasting, nutrient preservation is dependent on the specific vegetable, oven temperature, and time. Nutrient access may go up with some vegetables and down in others.

Frying is always the least healthy, but oftentimes the best tasting. It's unrealistic to expect people to look up the best method for cooking vegetables. When possible, default to microwaving and steaming with the shortest time, remembering that the most important thing is to eat a variety—of lots—of fruits and vegetables via any method of cooking.

Cooking Oils

Choosing cooking oils can be quite confusing because so many oils have been demonized. In reality, one should select oils that are unsaturated because they are healthier than saturated oils. Saturated and unsaturated fats are discussed in Chapter 5. Additionally, mix up the oils you use because different oils have different benefits. With respect to olive oil, this type of oil is part of the healthy Mediterranean diet. "Extra virgin" on olive oil labels means that the oil is not refined, and therefore a higher quality than oil that has been refined. You have to be aware because a 2015 National Consumers League tested 11 different olive oils in the United States and found several that failed to meet the "extra virgin" claim.

Vegetable oils come from plant sources. The healthfulness depends on its original plant source and most are a blend of canola, corn, soybean, safflower, palm, and sunflower. Canola oil is derived from the rapeseed plant, so it is highly processed and contains fewer nutrients overall. In addition to being in food, rapeseed oil is also used as a lubricant and in alternative fuels. While coconuts are plants, coconut oil is not classified as a vegetable oil because it is primarily saturated fat. It tastes good, though, so a little every now and then isn't horrible. Here is a table listing some common oils with key characteristics.

Common Oils with Key Characteristics

Oil	Key Characteristics
Avocado	Monounsaturated and polyunsaturated fat High in vitamin E Good for stir fry and high-heat cooking
Canola	Highly processed Unsaturated fat Good for high-heat cooking
Coconut	High saturated fat Good for frying
Flaxseed	Unsaturated fat Rich in omega-3 fatty acids Not good for cooking
Olive	Monounsaturated and polyunsaturated fat Polyphenols for health
Peanut	High monosaturated fat content Rich in vitamin E Good for cooking

Oil	Key Characteristics
Safflower	Unsaturated fat Rich in vitamin E Good for cooking
Sesame	Monounsaturated and polyunsaturated fat Good for cooking
Sunflower	Unsaturated fat High in vitamin E Omega-6 fatty acids Good for cooking
Vegetable	Unsaturated fat
Walnut oil	Unsaturated fat Good ration of omega-6 and omega-3 fatty acids Not good for cooking

Superfoods

What in the world are "superfoods"? It's a term that gets tossed around in popular newsfeeds. Superfood is not a scientific term, but it is a marketing term. And it's now included in the Merriam-Webster dictionary. So, if it's in the dictionary and it's making headlines, it's time to explain it. According to the dictionary, a superfood is a nutrient-rich food considered to be especially beneficial for health and well-being. The Harvard Health Blog even lists 10 superfoods, including berries, fish, leafy greens, nuts, olive oil, whole grains, yogurt, cruciferous vegetables, legumes, and tomatoes. It's important to be aware, because even Harvard Health notes that "no single food—not even a superfood—can offer all the nutrition, health benefits, and energy we need to nourish ourselves. The 2015–2020 U.S. Dietary Guidelines recommend healthy eating patterns, combining healthy choices from across all food groups—while paying attention to calorie limits." That said, many of these *superfoods* offer benefits, and instead of *superfoods*, scientists use the phrase "functional foods that supply phytochemicals."

Functional foods, or *nutraceuticals*, contain health-giving additives that have medicinal benefit. *Phytochemicals* are non-nutritive, biologically active compounds found in plants. Many nutraceuticals and phytochemicals are currently under study for their potential to prevent or treat diseases. An entire book can be written about these superfoods, so it's beyond the scope of this chapter. What's important to know is that there is evidence for and against some of the heavily-touted superfoods so it's important to consume them in moderation. Hype doesn't mean healthy. We'll turn our attention now to some of these so-called superfoods.

Yogurt

Yogurt is a semisolid food prepared from milk that has been fermented by adding bacteria. It is often flavored with fruit and added sweeteners. Yogurt has been eaten for hundreds of years across many cultures. Yogurt is rich in many nutrients, namely protein, calcium, B vitamins, phosphorus, magnesium, and potassium. Because it is a dairy product, vitamin D is usually added to help with the absorption of calcium. Its high protein content has been linked to appetite and weight control. Bacterial strains in yogurt differ depending on the manufacturer, but common strains are *Bifidobacteria* and *Lactobacillus*. These bacteria are important probiotics, which boost digestive health (reducing bloating, diarrhea, and constipation) and have other functions discussed in Chapter 2. Studies have also found that yogurt boosts heart health, increases the "good" HDL cholesterol, and decreases blood pressure.

That all sounds fine and dandy. However, yogurt is a milk product and has ill effects on people who are lactose intolerant or have a milk allergy. Lactose is milk sugar, which requires the enzyme, lactase, to be broken down. People who are lactose intolerant lack this enzyme, so if they consume yogurt, they could suffer abdominal pain and diarrhea. Milk also contains two proteins, casein and whey, that some people are allergic to. If people with a milk allergy consume casein or whey, they could react with hives or with much more serious life-threatening consequences such as anaphylaxis.

Blueberries

Blueberries are another highly touted superfood. Are blueberries a superfood? Numerous studies are showing that blueberries demonstrate a wide array of health-enhancing benefits. Blueberries contain plant pigments known as flavonoids that act as antioxidants. You may see the terms *flavonoids* and *flavonols* used interchangeably. Scientifically, flavonols are a class of flavonoids. For our purposes, the term flavonoids will be used as these are the substances studied for their effects on the body. As a group, they have anti-oxidative, anti-inflammatory, anti-mutagenic, and anti-carcinogenic properties. Antioxidants counter free radicals, the harmful, yet natural, byproducts of cellular metabolism. To combat free radicals and their subsequent damage, diets rich in foods that have antioxidants are important. Free radicals contribute to cancer and other age-related diseases. Benefits from eating a diet rich in blueberries include lowering blood cholesterol, lowering blood pressure, halting cataract progression, suppressing some types of cancer cell growth, and improving memory and brain function. Like cranberries, blueberries combat urinary tract infections by preventing bacteria from adhering to the lining of the urinary tract. Blueberries also contain anthocyanin, another flavonoid, that has anti-diabetes effects by improving insulin sensitivity and lowering blood glucose (sugar) levels. Blueberries may also reduce muscle soreness by diminishing inflammation and oxidative stress. The medicinal effects of blueberries have been known for centuries, and native peoples shared their knowledge of these fruits with Plymouth, Massachusetts, colonists. Thus, blueberries appear to be nutritious, quite healthy, and pack a lot of bang for the buck whether they are eaten fresh or frozen.

Cranberries

Cranberries are related to blueberries and have similar health benefits related to their antioxidant compounds. These bioactive compounds found primarily in cranberry skins are quercetin, myricetin, peonidin, ursolic acid, and A-type proanthocyanidins (condensed tannins). Cranberries, cranberry juice, and cranberry supplements may reduce the risk of urinary tract infections (UTIs), but they do not treat an established infection. They pack a nutritious punch, but are bitter, so sugar is often added to cranberries. Moreover, since most of the antioxidants are found in the berry skins, the bioactive compounds are reduced in the juice or in processed cranberry products.

Tomatoes

Botanically speaking, tomatoes are fruits, but they are prepared and typically eaten like a vegetable. They are great sources of vitamin C, vitamin K, folate, and potassium. Tomatoes also contain the antioxidants lycopene, beta carotene (the body converts this to vitamin A), chlorogenic acid, and the flavonoid, naringenin. Studies have shown that eating tomatoes may reduce the risk of heart disease and some cancers. In general, the redder the tomato, the more lycopene it contains. Generally, we think of raw food sources as containing the most nutrients. However, processed tomato products contain more lycopene than fresh tomatoes because during processing, water is lost, thus the lycopene is concentrated. When processing involves heat, the lycopene also becomes more bioavailable, meaning the body can readily use it. Because tomatoes are often picked before they are ripe, they undergo a commercial ripening process which entails spraying them with artificial ethylene gas. When tomatoes ripen naturally, they produce the gaseous hormone ethylene. Commercial ripening may make the tomatoes look more palatable, but the process inhibits natural flavor development, so commercially ripened tomatoes lack the flavor of fresh-off-the vine tomatoes.

Dark Chocolate

Dark chocolate. Yum. In addition to its 600 calories, a 3.5-ounce bar of this slightly bitter, deep brown chocolate is an excellent source of fiber, iron, magnesium, copper, and manganese, plus antioxidants. It also contains a little caffeine and theobromine. Eating 600 calories of dark chocolate is not something you should do daily, however.

Like blueberries and cranberries, the flavonoids in dark chocolate are powerful antioxidants, while the caffeine and theobromine are both stimulants. Theobromine is also found in tea and is a byproduct of natural caffeine metabolism in the liver.

Dark chocolate may improve blood flow through the arteries, which in turn lowers blood pressure. How does it lower blood pressure? The flavonoids stimulate the production of nitric oxide (NO) in arterial linings. Nitric oxide causes the blood vessels to relax and blood flow resistance to decrease, thereby easing blood flow through the cardiovascular system. Viagra, the drug used to treat erectile dysfunction, also works the same way by enhancing the nitric-oxide mediated vasodilation. Basically, it opens up the tubes within blood vessels and allows more blood to flow through without resistance.

Although its name suggests that there is bromine in theobromine, there is none. The term theobromine (*theo* = god + *broma* = food + *ine* = alkaloid) is derived from *Theobroma* the genus name of the cacao tree, *Theobroma cacao*. The amount of theobromine in chocolate varies, with dark chocolate containing higher concentrations than milk chocolate.

Many of us likely know that we shouldn't feed chocolate to dogs. One reason that dogs—and other animals besides humans—should not eat chocolate is because dogs metabolize the theobromine slower than humans, causing more to remain in the bloodstream. This leads to theobromine poisoning, which can cause death. In 2014, four American black bears died from theobromine-induced heart failure after eating chocolate and doughnuts used as bait in New Hampshire. In 2011, a black bear cub died the same way in Michigan.

Coffee, Caffeine, Tea and Theophylline

Ahh, a steaming cup of coffee, that hot drink made from the roasted and ground seed (coffee bean) of a shrub. Are there health benefits from the brewed drink? Like everything else cited as something that should be consumed in moderation, this is also true about coffee. Two cups of java per day has been linked to lowering one's risk for diabetes, Parkinson's disease, liver cancer, and heart failure. The balancing act is tricky and relies on individual physiology and whatever constitutes as "standard cup."

Caffeine is a stimulant to the central nervous system. As such, it is the world's most widely consumed psychoactive drug. It'll provide a little boost or the so-called "pick-me-up." Too much caffeine, though, increases blood pressure, causes insomnia, increases irritability, increases digestive distress, and leads to polyuria (excessive urination).

While caffeine shouldn't be consumed by people with heart arrhythmias, caffeine is used as therapy in preterm infants. In premature babies, caffeine is quite effective in treating apnea (temporary stoppage of breathing), intermittent hypoxemia (low oxygen in the blood), and it aids removal from mechanical ventilation (breathing machine).

Theophylline is related to caffeine and is a bitter compound found in tea leaves. It is the isomer of theobromine, meaning it has the same formula as theobromine, but the atoms in the molecule are arranged differently. As a drug, theophylline is used to treat chronic obstructive pulmonary disease (COPD) and asthma because it relaxes bronchial smooth muscles in breathing passages, allowing greater air flow. As a compound related to caffeine, it has similar effects of caffeine including being a stimulant and increasing the force and rate of heart contractions. Let's compare and contrast here.

Substance	Effects
Caffeine	• metabolized into theophylline and theobromine • stimulant
Theophylline	• relaxes bronchial smooth muscles • stimulates force and rate of heart muscle contractions
Theobromine	• improves blood flow • stimulates force and rate of heart muscle contractions

Coffee contains more caffeine than tea, but caffeine in both instances is a stimulant, giving you a jolt of energy and possibly that feeling of being "wired"—a ramped up nervous system. A cup of coffee has 100–300 mg of caffeine and a cup of tea has 20–60 mg. Both coffee and tea have antioxidants, while tea also contains the amino acid L-theanine, which increases brain wave activity and brain function.

Coffee does not prevent dementia. If you've heard that it does, there is still no research to back it up. A recent umbrella review, which is research that combines multiple analyses to provide a summary, found that drinking three to four cups of coffee per day did provide more benefit than harm, but it didn't prevent cognitive decline.

While coffee won't protect you from dementia, coffee can stimulate your bowels after surgery. A common side effect of sedation is that the drugs used to put you to sleep also cause your intestinal tract to rest as well. Drinking coffee does seem to stimulate post-operative bowel function. Since caffeine is a stimulant, it stimulates muscles along the digestive tract, which can help with constipation. Caffeine is also dehydrating, and dehydration can lead to constipation. So, if you drink coffee for stimulating your bowels, be sure to drink plenty of water along with the cup of coffee.

Red Wine

Oxidative stress is the burden placed on the body as a result of free radicals. One cause of widespread inflammation in the body is free radicals. As more is learned about disease and disease risk, much of it is linked to inflammation, a topic discussed in the next chapter. Antioxidants combat free radicals and lower oxidative stress. Chronic inflammation can be treated through diet, stress reduction, exercise, and red wine. You read that correctly.

Resveratrol, a compound in red wine, has antioxidant and anti-inflammatory properties and is currently under investigation for possible anti-cancer effects. Some studies show more promise than others: one study found that consuming one glass of red wine daily significantly reduced inflammatory markers, while another study found only slight reductions. Individual genetics or other factors not yet known may play a role in red wine's ability to affect inflammation.

Other studies showed that red wine conferred heart benefits. For example, drinking one glass per day may reduce blood pressure in people who already have hypertension. It may also assist blood pressure medication in further lowering blood pressure. The key compound for heart health seems to be polyphenol antioxidants. (If you are not a fan of red wine, kale also contains high levels of polyphenols.) Yet, drinking excessive alcohol adversely affects heart health and can lead to liver cirrhosis and heart disease. Recent studies have linked red wine consumption to promoting growth of beneficial gut bacteria, a topic discussed later in the book. In all, moderation seems to be key.

Cinnamon

Cinnamon is an ancient spice dating to 2000 BCE that is made from the bark of a Southeast Asian tree from the genus *Cinnamomum*. There are several species of the tree, yielding different types of this aromatic spice. The two main types are Cassia and Ceylon. Cassia is the most common type in the United States while Ceylon cinnamon is sold elsewhere. Its role in lowering LDL-cholesterol and HDL-cholesterol has not been substantiated in the professional literature.

Because cinnamon is loaded with antioxidants, it does have anti-inflammatory properties. We know that lowering inflammation lowers the risk of disease. Some studies show that when taken at a dosage of one-half to two teaspoons per day, cinnamon may lower fasting blood sugar levels in people who have diabetes. Other studies are not able to confirm this health benefit. This appears to be a case of needing to wait for more evidence. What we do know is that the popular viral Internet "cinnamon challenge" in which people videoed themselves eating a spoonful of ground cinnamon in under 60 seconds without drinking anything is a health risk not worth taking for a few moments of fame. Besides choking and gagging, this risky practice is dangerous to the lungs and can cause respiratory failure. Don't do this at home or anywhere ever.

Turmeric and Curcumin

Turmeric, a member of the ginger family, is an aromatic spice that gives curry its yellow color. It has been used in Indian cooking for thousands of years and is touted as having medicinal purposes. The active ingredient in turmeric that appears to be an anti-inflammatory agent is curcumin. Research in clinical trials have found no support for clinical use. Despite the $150 million U.S. government supported research into curcumin at the National Center for Complementary and Integrative Health, no health benefit has been found.

Complementary and Alternative Medicine, Integrative Health and the Placebo Response

Time to turn our attention to alternative/complementary/integrative medicine, because nutrition information is one area in which the fakes outpace the reals. The great expense of new, modern pharmaceutical medications, as well as instrumentation and surgical costs, and the uncertainty of the future of current health care programs and coverage have caused many Americans (nearly half of all U.S. adults) to look outside the conventional medical health system. Many are looking toward other means of complementary and alternative treatment for their health care.

What is complementary and alternative medicine? Complementary medicine is the utilization of practices in conjunction with mainstream medicine while alternative medicine is used instead of mainstream medicine. Both include treatments and practices that lack scientific plausibility or have not been studied enough to know for sure whether a treatment or supplement works. The names sound fancy and make it seem like this stuff is real, but many therapies and supplements have been untested and/or shown to be ineffective. We hear much about herbal remedies used for mood disorders and treatment for a number of medical problems. There's even a journal devoted to such medicine, *Journal of Alternative and Complementary Medicine*. In fact, this journal is advertised as a peer-reviewed medical journal and the official journal of the Society of Acupuncture Research. The Osher Collaborate for Integrative Medicine partners with them. Here's where it gets tricky. The Osher Collaborate for Integrative Medicine is an international group of seven academic centers funded by the Bernard Osher Foundation to study, teach, and practice integrative medicine. Those seven centers are respected in the area of science and include University of California (San Francisco), Harvard University, Karolinska Institutet, Northwestern University, Vanderbilt University, University of Miami, and University of Washington. The group has a section on Integrative Nutrition, which focuses on whole foods and a whole-person approach to nutrition and health. Registered dietitians staff the facilities. Per their website, the research findings are consistent with mainstream science:

> Research has found positive effects of nutrition intervention on many medical conditions in various age groups. This has been particularly true in the areas of overweight and obesity, diabetes, and heart health. Studies demonstrate that the inclusion of nutrition intervention and counseling by a registered dietitian as part of a healthcare team resulted in significant improvements in weight and body mass index, blood sugar markers, blood pressure, and serum lipids. Additionally, nutrition intervention has shown a positive effect on cancer survivorship and tolerance to treatment, improved inflammatory markers in autoimmune conditions, and improved behavior and attention in children with neurodevelopmental issues who have underlying food intolerances.

The next statement on their website is "Payment Information." Many ancillary treatments and therapies, for the most part, have not been fully scientifically checked, rigorously tested, and evaluated to date. That's not to say that they don't work; it's to say that we should view them with some skepticism as there is not enough known about them yet. Rigorous testing using the scientific method must occur.

The effectiveness of many practices is still greatly debatable, and there may be both beneficial as well as harmful effects. Induced harmful effects is particularly true with a great variety of herbals, resulting from their excessive and unregulated use. There may be allergic reactions due to toxic impurities and incorrectly mixed herbs as well as interactions with prescription drugs. Yet, very few people dispute their potential significance as the treatments are widely used and the public appears to be "positively convinced" of their beneficial effects, even though they are not abandoning conventional medicine entirely. Belief in healing powers of herbs and supplements cannot be discounted because the placebo response—beneficial effect of something that cannot be attributed to the properties of the herb itself—is real.

In 1998, the National Institutes of Health turned its Office of Alternative Medicine (OAM), then a very small enterprise, into a full-strength federal agency and called it the National Center for Complementary and Alternative Medicine (NCCAM). The NCCAM is now known as the National Center for Complementary and Integrative Health (NCCIH) and is part of the 27 institutes comprising the National

Institutes of Health (NIH) within the federally-funded Department of Health and Human Services. It funds research in five main areas: whole medical systems, mind-body medicine, biologically-based practices, manipulative and body-based practices, and energy therapies.

Large clinical trials are being designed to assess the merits of popular therapies. For example, there are studies evaluating the use, risks, and benefits of the supplements glucosamine and chondroitin sulfate in the treatment of osteoarthritis; others study the use of acupuncture to ease arthritis pain; some are looking at the use of selenium and vitamin E to prevent prostate cancer; and many are assessing the ability of Ginkgo biloba to preserve mental function as we age. The list is virtually endless.

Nevertheless, there are many skeptics who fear that science-based medicine may suffer because the National Center for Complementary and Integrative Health studies alternative and complementary practices. Scientific journals, including *Science*, and other publications have been extremely critical of NCCIH because they fund studies not based in science but rather founded in politics and other non-meritorious agendas. Clinical practice may be revolutionized as more information is made available through intense research, trials, and evaluations; and we may be looking forward to a new form of integrative medicine in modern health care.

Like weight loss diets, supplements, and herbal remedies, alternative therapies are big business. Why are some therapies helpful even when there is no scientific evidence to support the treatment? That is, they work even though there's no underlying scientific explanation. The answer lies in the placebo response/placebo effect. A placebo is a harmless pill, medicine, procedure, or touch that is prescribed for its psychological benefit or its suggestive effect. Without medicinal properties, a placebo should have no physiological effect. In fact, before drugs are marketed to the general public, they are tested using placebos. In drug testing, an inert compound that is identical in appearance to a new drug being tested in experimental research is administered to test subjects so that the researcher can distinguish between drug action and suggestive effect of the new drug under study. For the most robust studies, the researcher does not know which drug is the treatment, nor which drug is the placebo. Interestingly, placebos can have just as great or greater effect than the actual drug, showing that our mind plays a huge role in making us better.

2

The GI Tract Is Not in the Army

Digestive System and Health

Anatomy and Physiology

If we are what we eat, how does food become us? It begins at the cellular level; thus, we must begin by outlining the levels of organization in the body. The smallest structural and functional unit of an organism is a cell. We cannot see most cells in our body without using a microscope. The exception is the oocyte, which is the egg cell released by female ovaries. While we can see this with the naked eye, it is still about the size of a grain of sand. Our cells are specialized and combine to form specific tissues, which in turn form particular organs that become parts of entire organ systems. Taken in total, cells, tissues, organs, and organ systems form organisms, which are us. See Figure 2.1 for the sequence.

Forming us and keeping us functioning involves the interplay of our 11 body systems. These eleven with some of their important structures include the following:

1. integumentary (skin and associated structures)
2. skeletal (bones, cartilages, and ligaments)
3. muscular (heart muscle, smooth muscle of internal organs, and skeletal muscles that attach to bones)
4. nervous (brain, spinal cord, and peripheral nerves)
5. endocrine (various glands and hormones)
6. cardiovascular (heart, blood, and blood vessels including arteries, veins, and capillaries)
7. lymphatic (lymph, lymph nodes, and immune cells)

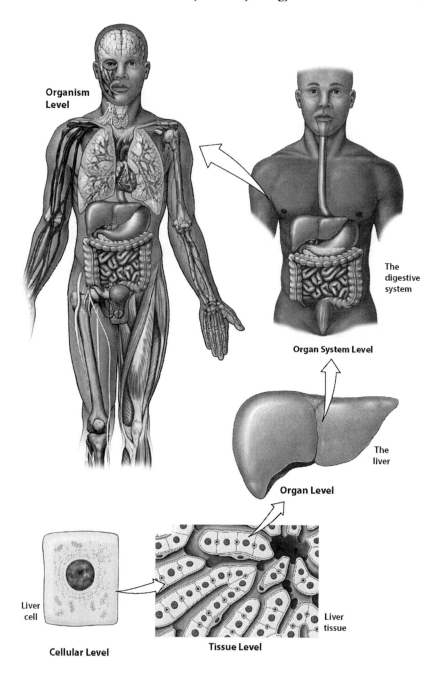

Figure 2.1 The levels of organization beginning with cells and ending with a human organism.

8. respiratory (nose, mouth, and lungs)
9. digestive (esophagus, stomach, intestines, and associated organs)
10. urinary (kidneys, ureters, bladder, and urethra)
11. reproductive (sex organs that vary between males and females)

In order to keep everything functioning, each cell requires energy, which is derived from the food we eat. At the center of it all is our DNA, the molecule that encodes our genetic makeup. DNA is found in the nucleus of the cell and long strands of DNA coil into the genes of our chromosomes. These genes contain instructions for making protein, which is used to make cells, the building blocks to tissue formation. Underlying all of this is what we eat because nutrition plays a role in our gene activities. An emerging field of study showing the connection between nutrition and genes is *nutritional genomics*, also called *nutrigenomics*. Through these emergent fields, we're learning more and more about what turns genes on and off and how nutrition at particular stages influences this gene activity. Nutrigenomics also studies the relationship between nutrition and overall health as it relates to our personal genetics.

Before we get too deep into the role of nutrition and genes, it makes sense to understand the structures and functions of the digestive system itself. As we just saw in the previous paragraph related to synonyms for nutritional genomics and nutrigenomics, names for the digestive system and its components becomes another lesson in vocabulary. Sometimes the digestive system is also called the gastrointestinal (GI) system, but this *gastrointestinal* assumes we're only discussing the stomach (*gastro*) and the intestines (*intestinal*). The term digestive *tract* is also used to describe the long continuous tube because in anatomy tract refers to a major passage. But the whole digestive system begins at the mouth and ends at the anus with many associated organs in between, whose jobs are to extract nutrients from the food we eat.

Think about eating a slice of pizza. Our body can't do anything with that slice of pizza until it is broken down into its component nutrients. Chewing begins this process, and in order for the body to use the component nutrients, they must be further broken down and processed into smaller molecules: Carbohydrates get broken down into simpler sugar; fats get broken down into fatty acids and glycerol; proteins get broken down into amino acids; while vitamins, minerals, and water are extracted from the food because these cannot be broken down any further. The breakdown units are either used, stored, or eliminated in feces (the fancy term for poop) and urine (pee).

This is where it gets a little complex because food-to-waste is not straightforward as it involves two separate body systems: digestive and urinary. Through the process of digestion, nutrients are absorbed into the bloodstream along the length of the digestive tract with some being absorbed in the stomach, but most being absorbed along the intestines. Urine is made when the kidneys filter blood while feces are made if the products of digestion haven't been absorbed by the blood. Basically, if the body can use the nutrients, they remain; otherwise, they are excreted as urine or feces. This demonstrates the delicate interplay between the two body systems.

Let's take a closer look at *how* the food and beverages we put in our mouths actually become components the body can use: digestion. Digestion is complicated and involves mechanical, chemical, and enzymatic processes that convert food to energy or waste. Primary organs involved with digestion are the mouth, esophagus, stomach, small intestine, large intestine, pancreas, liver, and gall bladder. Review the chart below that identifies the digestive organs with some key functions and refer back to it if you need a refresher. Then, look at Figure 2.2 that shows key organs of the digestive system.

Digestive Organs and Some Key Functions

Organs	Key Functions
Mouth	Opening through which we take in food; beginning of the digestive system where mechanical digestion starts by chewing and chemical digestion begins by enzymes secreted in the mouth
Esophagus	Muscular tube connecting the mouth with the stomach; about 10 inches long
Stomach	Muscular sac between the esophagus and small intestine; involved with mechanical (churning) and chemical (enzymes and hydrochloric acid) digestion of food; about 10–11 inches long and 3–4 inches wide
Small intestine	Muscular tube between the stomach and the large intestine; nutrients are absorbed here; about 20 feet long
Large intestine	Muscular tube between the small intestine and the anus (opening to the exterior); absorbs fluids and electrolytes (minerals); stores feces prior to defecation; about 5 feet long

Organs	Key Functions
Pancreas	Gland nestled between the stomach and first fold of the small intestine; connected to small intestine through the pancreatic duct; secretes the hormones insulin and glucagon; secretes enzymes for digestion; about 6 inches long
Liver	Largest gland in the body; secretes bile for fat breakdown, receives recently absorbed nutrients, detoxifies drugs; important in fat, carbohydrate, and protein metabolism; stores glycogen; weighs about 2.2–4.4 pounds and the dimensions vary with body size
Gallbladder	Organ tucked into a shallow depression below the right lobe of the liver; stores bile; about 3–4 inches in length and 2 inches in diameter

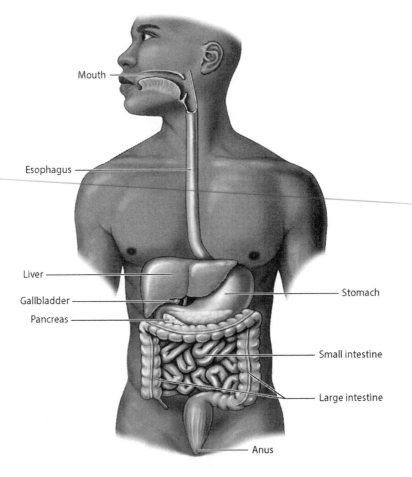

Figure 2.2 Key organs of the digestive system.

Food processing involves four basic stages: ingestion, digestion, absorption, and elimination. During ingestion, we eat food or drink liquids through our mouths. Teeth and jaws grind up the food, and we begin salivating. Just putting stuff in our mouths—or smelling something really good—automatically begins saliva production.

Our teeth begin mechanical digestion, the process whereby food is physically broken down into smaller particles in the mouth by chewing and this continues further in the stomach by churning. The fancy term for chewing is *mastication*. This is a funny term, and I often relay a distasteful story (pun intended) told to me as an undergraduate student sitting in a lecture hall of a couple hundred hungry minds. It goes something like this. A wizened anatomy and physiology professor was lecturing on this very topic, introducing key terms, which we diligently wrote in our Trapper Keepers using our chic Bic 4-color retractable ballpoint pens. This sage on the stage chuckled and told us, "After masticating, you don't have to wash your hands." We dutifully laughed. Some got the reference; others did not. Throughout my career, it's always been a judgment call as to whether or not to tell that story. In today's culture, it's probably best left to academic circles and this book. Looking back, I think this guy was more than a little twisted. Might explain why he still lived with his mom.

Chewing is a critical piece of eating and having working teeth is important throughout life. When we are missing teeth, it is more difficult to chew food, making digestion harder. Missing teeth also leads to bone loss in the jaw because we need the physical stimulation of teeth biting down on hard surfaces to stimulate bone cells to form new bone. Bone building and breaking down, known as bone cycling, is a life-long process. This is one reason why people who wear dentures oftentimes have to get them refitted throughout life.

Teeth, chewing, and jaw structure are rooted in evolution. In human anatomy and physiology, we have a saying that "form follows function." It means that the form of a body structure (anatomy) is related to its function (physiology). Two examples related to form following function involve the mouth. The first example is forming a rounded mass called a *bolus*. Because square pegs don't do well with round holes, we need to form a structure that can pass easily through the cylindrical esophagus, the passageway between the mouth and the stomach. As food mixes with saliva, a bolus of chewed up food forms.

The second example relates to tooth shape and size and demonstrates the purpose of each type. Teeth are also good predictors of diet types. Foods eaten by our long-ago ancestors, along with the processing of foods by fire and tools, affected the evolution of our jaws and teeth. If we look at our jaws and teeth, we have two jaws and 32 teeth. The immovable upper jaw is the maxilla, and the movable lower jaw is the mandible. Four main types of teeth are found within the jaws: incisors, canines (cuspids), pre-molars (bicuspids), and molars, which are the biggest teeth we have. If you know the derivation of each term, you can figure out what it looks like and what it does. The word *incisor* comes from the Latin, *incis*, meaning *cutter*. Cuspids are teeth with a single point, derived from the Latin word *cuspis* meaning *point*. Bicuspids (*bi* = two) have two cusps. The word *molar* is derived from the Latin word *molaris*, which means *millstone*. Millstones were circular stones used for grinding grain.

We have eight incisors (four on the upper maxilla and four on the lower mandible) front and center for biting off food. The four sharp, pointy canines (two on top and two on bottom) tear food and the eight pre-molars (four on top and four on bottom) and 12 molars (which include four wisdom teeth) have flat surfaces that are used for tearing, crushing, and grinding during chewing.

Looking through an evolutionary lens, we know that human wisdom teeth once had a function when human mouths were bigger, and our pre-cooking diets revolved around eating tough, fibrous foods. The bigger mouths gave us room for the extra four molars, which also replaced teeth lost from chewing hardy foodstuffs.

Across the animal kingdom, the dentition (*dent* = tooth) pattern is replicated in that there are incisors, canines, bicuspids, and molars. If we look at our closest relative, chimpanzees, we see that like us, they have the same number of teeth and in the same order. They also have baby teeth that are lost when the adult teeth grow in. There is one major difference: chimps have much larger, carnivorous-sized canines than we do. Why would this be if chimps are primarily plant-based eaters? The reason is threat. Big canines can be intimidating and can demonstrate to would-be enemies that "I have big teeth that can bite you." Most animals use their canine teeth for fighting. For interest, compare human jaws with jaws of carnivorous animals like your dog and cat. In both dogs and cats, their canines are much bigger than in humans. Again, big canines warn predators and threats to stay away from my bite, which will hurt. While the different types of teeth are the same in dogs, cats, humans, and chimps, the number and arrangement vary. Dogs have 42 teeth, 20 in the upper jaw and 22 in the lower jaw; and cats have 30 teeth,

16 in the upper jaw and 14 in the lower jaw. The variation is a result of evolution and purposes between early herbivores (humans) and carnivores (dogs and cats). Humans, dogs, and cats today are omnivores, eating both plants and animals.

The next step in converting food to usable particles is chemical digestion. During chemical digestion, enzymes break down food into smaller subunits. Enzymes are substances, usually proteins, that catalyze (speed up) biochemical reactions, that are not used up in the process, but they can be unfolded and inactivated by heat or chemical changes. This is called denaturing, and in the body, denaturing is permanent. For an example you can see, denaturing is what happens when you cook an egg: the protein in the egg white changes from a liquid to a solid, and once it does that, there is no going back to the slimy egg white. This is one reason why we need to continually create new enzymes and therefore a reason why we need vitamins, which act as co-enzymes. Enzymes are produced by the body and some control reactions within cells while others, such as those of digestion, control reactions outside cells. Our cells are enclosed by a membrane that acts like a semi-permeable seal with stuff inside and stuff outside.

Chemical digestion also begins in the mouth with enzymes in saliva (spit) and continues throughout the digestive tract with other enzymes added in the stomach and small intestine. A clue that something is an enzyme is the suffix, -ase, which means *enzyme*.

Now, if you'd like to try an experiment at home, place a dry saltine cracker on your tongue. Within seconds, you'll notice that you begin to salivate and may taste a little sweetness. The reason is because the enzyme in saliva, called *salivary amylase*, begins breaking down the carbohydrate—a sugar—in the cracker. Fun, right? Since digestion breaks down food into its usable components, molecules like carbohydrates are broken down into simpler sugars. Fats are broken down into fatty acids and glycerol. Proteins are broken down into amino acids. And vitamins and minerals are extracted from the foods. Your body *"knows"* what to do with these smaller particles.

So far, we've discussed ingestion and digestion, the first two stages. The next two stages are absorption and elimination. In the stomach, acid helps break down food and nutrients, forming a pasty mixture of gastric juices and partly digested food called *chyme*. This chyme gets passed into the intestines for absorption. Absorption happens when water and nutrients from digested food enter the bloodstream along the intestines, which are wrapped with capillaries (teeny tiny blood vessels).

Alcohol and some drugs can be absorbed by the stomach, but most food absorption occurs in the intestines.

The pasty chyme moves along the length of the intestines—from the stomach's exit to the body exterior—by a process called *peristalsis*. Think of the entire intestinal tract as one long smooth muscle that contracts in waves, much like squeezing toothpaste from a tube, pushing the chyme along. As it moves through the tube, nutrients we need are absorbed by capillaries surrounding the intestines. The food we eat does little good until those nutrients get into the bloodstream where they can be delivered to the body's cells. Broken down food and water are absorbed along the length of the small intestine, a tube about 20 feet long. Only water is absorbed by the five-foot-long large intestine. Physiologists would consider this an overly simplified explanation, but for our purpose, it totally suffices. If you'd like to learn more, take an anatomy and physiology (A&P) course or buy an A&P book.

Here's an interesting question, though. If the small intestine is roughly 20 feet long, and the large intestine is about five feet long, why would the longer intestine be labeled "small" while the shorter intestine is called "long"? It has to do with the size of the lumen (interior) of the intestines. The intestines are like twisting and turning crazy straws whose hollow interior—the lumen—remains open. The large intestine's lumen is wider than the small intestine's lumen, hence it's called the *large intestine.*

From an evolutionary perspective, the intestine length has changed over time, and the length of our intestines is shorter than in the chimpanzee and orangutan. It has been suggested that our intestines got smaller so that more energy could be expended toward increased brain size. Another suggestion is that cooking reduced the need for increased intestine length because early humans could extract more nutrients from food that had been broken down or partially broken down through cooking; thus, less metabolic energy was required to extract nutrients from the food. An important point here to know is that intestinal tissue is metabolically active tissue, so it requires energy from food to operate effectively. Yes, the act of digesting expends energy. While food is being broken down along the length of the intestines, energy is required for this process.

Elimination is the last stage of food processing. Any undigested food and excess water forms feces. While both feces and urine are wastes, they are distinctly different biological entities. Here's the difference between feces and urine: Feces is waste matter made up of undigested food that never enters body cells, while urine contains wastes produced by the body's cells.

The large intestine is the last section that continues to draw water out of the feces as it is forming. This water is retained by the bloodstream; and if the excess water isn't drawn off, diarrhea results. Formed feces exit the body through the anus.

You might be thinking, "Hey, if the GI tract is one long tube, can't I just do a little experiment to see *how* long it is by swallowing a really long piece of dental floss and waiting to see if it comes out my butt?" The dumb answer is, "Well, yes, you can." The smart answer is, "Yes, it's possible, but it could also kill you, so don't do it." After all, if you're a pet owner, you may have experienced something similar. Who hasn't been surprised by a little tinsel hanging from your dog's behind a day or two after putting up the Christmas tree? If so, you likely helped Spot remove the dangling tinfoil by gently tugging until the poo-covered silver was safely extracted. Consider two things about this scenario: One, this tugging likely did no harm because the tinsel was short. Two, this tugging maybe did some harm because the tinsel was longer than expected and could have cut through the twists and turns of the intestines causing internal bleeding. It is for this last reason that you should never try your own version of butt flossing.

Hormones

We've gone through the organs of digestion, now it's time to add a little more function to those organs. Human digestive physiology is complicated because it interacts with so many other systems plus human behavior. We're learning more and more about the interactions of body systems, human behavior, and the various axes linking these systems together. We're also learning more about eating in moderation. One area ripe with study is the interaction of hormones with the body. Hormones are chemical messengers that are released into the bloodstream and exert their effects at a site distant from where they were originally released, or they are released into tissue fluids and exert their effects locally. Some hormones do something else and interact with the nervous system to influence whether we feel hungry or full.

How do we know when we are full (satiated)? Good question, because we often eat when we are not hungry. Satiety is that feeling of being satisfied. In our brains, we have a rather small area referred to as the *satiety center*, located specifically within the hypothalamus, which is another small gland. This part of the brain sends signals to our conscious self that we are full and don't need to eat any more. The hypothalamus also does much more than house our satiety center—it also controls body temperature, mood, and motivation. For example, on a normal day, when you are thirsty you drink one glass of water, you don't drink 20 glasses of water. You knew you were thirsty because water receptors in the brain called *osmoreceptors* sent a signal telling you this. You drank a glass of water and were sated. You *knew* this because stretch receptors from your stomach sent another signal back up to your brain telling you this. Yet, because the hypothalamus also controls mood, eating could make us feel good, so we eat when we are not hungry. So far so good?

Having said that, there are other significant hormones including insulin, ghrelin, leptin, and glucagon that influence numerous aspects of human digestion. Insulin is a hormone secreted by cells in the pancreas. To be scientifically specific, insulin is a polypeptide hormone secreted by the beta cells in the pancreas. This is good to know in case you're ever playing trivia or watching television commercials for diabetes drugs that mention beta cells.

The pancreas is an organ that looks like a flat piece of gyro meat and is located close to the stomach and small intestine. In fact, it is strategically located within the first fold of the small intestine, known as the duodenum, which is the connector tube between the stomach and the rest of the small intestine. By strategically located, I mean that once partially digested food—the so-called chyme—empties from the stomach, it enters the duodenum. At this point, acidic chyme needs more chemicals to help process it. Those chemicals come from the pancreas.

Pancreatic insulin promotes glucose (the body's sugar) use, protein synthesis, and the formation and storage of lipids (fats). Obviously, it has various important roles! Insulin helps regulate the amount of glucose in the bloodstream by helping glucose move from the bloodstream into the cells. This is a topic that trips up some people, so think about it thusly: Imagine having a straw full of water and Skittles where the water represents the bloodstream with dissolved substances like glucose and the Skittles represent cells. Our cells are surrounded by fluid and in this case, that fluid is blood. If the glucose within the blood can't get into the cells, it doesn't do any good out in the bloodstream. Cells require glucose *in them*, not around them, to function.

Our second hormone is ghrelin (pronounced grel'in). Ghrelin is a gut-brain hormone that is produced mainly in the stomach (gut) and hypothalamus in the brain. Ghrelin stimulates appetite. During fasting or when blood glucose levels are low, ghrelin levels increase; during feeding, ghrelin levels decrease. This is known as negative feedback or internal counteracting. However, in people who are chronically obese, ghrelin levels are decreased, thereby interfering with negative feedback mechanisms. The association between ghrelin and obesity is quite complex and involves other factors as well, which are actively being studied.

Ghrelin can also be given to people to induce a feeling of hunger or to increase appetite. For example, in cancer patients who have lost their appetite, ghrelin can be given to stimulate the appetite. It's interesting to note that blood levels of ghrelin are measurably higher in patients who have lost weight through dietary measures.

The third hormone, leptin, also plays a role in appetite. Leptin is secreted by fat cells. It acts on the hypothalamus to curb appetite and to increase energy expenditure while also regulating fat storage in the body. Leptin levels are 40 percent higher in women than in men and increase to 50 percent higher just before girls have their first menstrual cycle. So there is a hike in leptin before a girl gets her first period. Fortunately, leptin returns to baseline levels after a few menstrual cycles. Leptin levels lower with fasting and they increase with inflammation. Thus, inflammation may have a role in obesity, and we know that chronic inflammation in the body plays a role in almost every major disease. All inflammation isn't bad though: when we cut our finger, the tissue becomes inflamed as blood containing important immune cells rushes to the site. Widespread chronic inflammation, however, is not good. Inflammation is discussed a little later in this chapter. Understanding leptin is quite complicated, though, because we now know that leptin also helps insulin transport glucose into fat cells. In studies of both lean and overweight people who were on weight-reduction diets and received daily injections of leptin, both lost weight that was proportionate to leptin dosage.

So what does this mean if you are trying to lose weight? We've heard over and over to cut calories, cut dietary fat, and eat smaller portions throughout the day. However, research is showing us this doesn't seem to work very well because there is an insulin versus leptin battle. The key to weight loss is to lower insulin. If we eat constantly, insulin levels go up. If we fast, insulin levels go down and so do leptin levels. What has been shown to work in cultures with the longest-lived people is to eat real, unprocessed food, more whole grains with lots of fruits and vegetables, and to practice time restricted eating or intermittent fasting. If you're hung up on the "intermittent fasting," simply not eating for 12-hour periods counts. What is a simple way to do that? If you get up at 7 a.m. every morning, then stop eating at 7 p.m. the night before. Fasting is also discussed in Chapter 9.

Research has also shown that people who eat in the morning and stop at mid-day have better blood pressure and insulin sensitivity. Other studies have shown that extending one's fasting time can help a person lose weight. This means that intermittent fasting and meal timing can help in weight management and metabolic health.

If you are generally healthy to begin with, you'll be okay with restricting eating time because of another pancreatic hormone known as glucagon. Glucagon comes from the alpha cells of the pancreas, and its job is to mobilize glycogen. Glucagon and glycogen sound a lot alike. Glycogen is the storage form of glucose (sugar). Time to take a break and look at a vocabulary chart:

Substance	Definition
Glucose	Sugar our cells use
Glycogen	Storage form of sugar; when we have too much glucose, the body changes it to another chemical called glycogen, which can be stored in our skeletal muscles and liver
Glucagon	Hormone that converts glycogen to glucose for use by our cells; it takes glycogen from storage, converts it to glucose, and places it in the bloodstream so our cells can access it

If the body has more sugar than it can use, it converts it to glycogen and stores it in the liver and skeletal muscles. Glucagon mobilizes glycogen from skeletal muscles and the liver and converts it back to glucose. Glucagon ensures that our blood level of glucose remains within an acceptable range. We don't want to starve our cells.

Nutrition and Upper Gastrointestinal Disorders

There are many disorders of the upper digestive tract, which consists of the mouth, esophagus, and stomach. Common ones requiring nutritional interventions are discussed here. Earlier, we discussed the importance of having teeth; but if chewing is difficult, weight loss and malnutrition could occur, so soft diets that are easy to chew and swallow are necessary. In addition to difficulty chewing, difficulty swallowing, termed *dysphagia*, can affect eating. Dysphagia can occur with aging, nervous system diseases, and stroke, but it doesn't always have an underlying disorder. Dysphagia can occur with common activities like talking, laughing, or lying down. Or dysphagia can happen if your mouth is dry, food is too hot, or if the medication "just won't go down." Nursing home dining rooms are places in which dysphagia is common. The reason is because aging-related dysphagia oftentimes results from anatomical changes in the neck region. As people age, osteoporosis becomes more prevalent, resulting in forward neck bending. Such changes make swallowing a little more difficult, and concomitant coughing is commonplace in older populations.

Another upper GI disorder is reflux esophagitis, a condition caused by gastric contents being regurgitated into the esophagus, causing esophageal inflammation with a burning sensation. The common term for this is *heartburn*. The esophagus feels like it is on fire because the gastric contents are acidic. When the ring of smooth muscle between the esophagus and stomach, known as the sphincter, does not close tightly, reflux esophagitis results. Antacids, which change the acidity in the stomach, can help alleviate the burning.

Another disorder affecting the stomach and esophagus is *hiatal hernia*, a protrusion of the stomach up through the esophageal hiatus (opening) of the diaphragm. From an anatomical perspective, from top to bottom, the esophagus enters the stomach through a natural hole in the diaphragm. The diaphragm is the dome-shaped muscle of breathing that looks like an umbrella covering the stomach. If the top part of the stomach protrudes through the opening, it creates an uncomfortable feeling because it is out of place. *Hernia* is the medical term for an organ that protrudes through another organ. People who have hiatal hernias are advised to eat smaller portions of food so that the stomach doesn't expand as much and to remain upright (instead of laying down) after eating.

Another common ailment is an ulcer, a sore that develops on the lining of the esophagus or stomach. With ulcers, the innermost layer of cells is eroded. The stomach has several layers, but the innermost layer of cells makes mucus, a slimy fluid that protects the stomach from its own acid. If that lining wears away, then the acid in the stomach burns a hole in the lining causing an ulcer. You might be wondering why the stomach has acid then. The acid is hydrochloric acid (HCl) and it plays a role in converting enzymes into other enzymes that are necessary for chemical digestion. Interestingly, a bacterium, *Helicobacter pylori*, is associated with causing many ulcers. This bacterium is found in 50–70 percent of people in Western countries, but only about 10 percent of people have stomach ulcers. In most cases, bacteria cannot live in our stomachs because of the low pH, which kills them. However, *Helicobacter pylori*, is an acidophile, a term that literally means "acid loving." (In case you were wondering why the words are in italics, it has to do with biological nomenclature: when writing the genus and species names of organisms, the genus name begins with a capital letter, the species name begins with a lowercase letter, and both terms are either italicized or underlined, depending on what your word processor can do.) The treatment for *Helicobacter pylori*-caused ulcers includes giving antibiotics to eradicate the infection. In 2005, Barry Marshall and Robin Warren were awarded the Nobel Prize in Physiology or Medicine for their work tying *Helicobacter pylori* with stomach ulcers. Prior to their discovery, many thought the majority of stomach ulcers were brought about by stress and were treated accordingly, including giving tranquilizing drugs or other medicines to relieve anxiety.

Nutrition and Lower Gastrointestinal Disorders

Disorders of the lower gastrointestinal tract include those involving the small intestine and large intestine. Lower GI disorders include diarrhea, constipation, diverticulosis, diverticulitis, and colitis. Diarrhea is a condition of loose, watery, frequent bowel movements. Its causes are varied and range from eating contaminated food or coming in contact with a virus, to parasites, and other bowel disorders. It can last from a day or two to weeks. Regardless of the cause, a person must make sure to drink plenty of fluids to replace water lost by the diarrhea to avoid dehydration and electrolyte imbalance. From a dietary perspective, it is treated with anti-diarrheal medication, a BRAT diet of *b*ananas, *r*ice, *a*pplesauce, and *t*oast, and possibly probiotics. Probiotics stimulate the growth of normal microorganisms, known as the intestinal flora, which would re-establish the good bacteria in the gut.

While daily bowel movements are perfectly normal, not having bowel movements for days is not normal. There will always be times in life when you are struck with either diarrhea or constipation, and for the most part, both can be treated at home. How many times per day a person has a bowel movement depends on many factors, and some people may feel constipated if they don't have a bowel movement daily or every other day. Yet, by medical standards, constipation is defined as having three or fewer bowel movements in a week and its causes aren't always due to underlying disease. Constipation is also characterized by hard, dry feces. It's the opposite of diarrhea, and like diarrhea, most people have experienced it. There are nutritional interventions for prevention, including eating lots of fruits, vegetables, and high-fiber food; drinking plenty of liquids; and getting exercise. These same preventions can also help treat the disorder.

Laxatives are also an effective treatment for constipation. There are four main types of laxatives: (1) bulk-forming, which are fiber supplements; (2) osmotic, which cause more water to move into the intestines; (3) stimulant, which stimulate the smooth muscle of the intestines to speed up movement; and (4) stool softeners, which cause more water to move into the feces thereby making them softer. Then there are prunes, the long-standing remedy for constipation. Prunes, prune juice, and "power pudding" (bran, applesauce, and prune juice) are known to relieve constipation. Some research shows that nutrients in prunes may prevent colon cancer, and can help control obesity, diabetes, and cardiovascular disease.

Other conditions of the intestines have similar sounding names, diverticulosis and diverticulitis, and you can't have one without the other. First, diverticula are abnormal pouches in the large intestine, and their presence creates the condition called *diverticulosis* (-osis = condition). If the diverticula become inflamed, the resulting condition is *diverticulitis* (-itis = inflammation). Surgery is sometimes necessary, but a high-fiber diet is routinely recommended.

The last section of the large intestine is called the *colon*. *Colitis* is inflammation of the colon lining. It is characterized by diarrhea, abdominal cramps, or constipation. Nutritional treatment follows the same protocol for diarrhea or constipation.

Inflammation

What we're learning about staying healthy involves keeping inflammation at bay. Inflammation is a normal physical response characterized by five so-called cardinal signs: redness, heat, swelling, pain, and loss of function. It appears that decreasing widespread inflammation in the body has an impact on our overall health and dietary measures can affect inflammation. As part of normal physiology, inflammation is part of the body's immune response to protect us from injury or disease. When you cut your finger, blood rushes to the wound site causing redness, heat, and swelling. Blood contains white blood cells and other substances that work to keep infection out and to begin healing. You feel pain because nerves have been activated, and once that happens, you stop doing the thing that caused you to get hurt. Generally speaking, inflammation is good. But prolonged, widespread inflammation is bad.

There are two types of inflammation: acute and chronic. The acute type is short-lived and resolves quickly. The finger-cutting example in the previous paragraph is a classic example of acute inflammation and is good as it speeds recovery and gets us back into action. Chronic inflammation is a prolonged inflammatory response and can have long-lasting effects. The response can occur with or without injury and if injury occurs, inflammation may not end after the injury has healed. For example, inflammation occurs when a person has a heart attack. If the person survives the heart attack, widespread (systemic) inflammation can still be a problem. Chronic inflammation is basically slow, long-term inflammation that sticks around after the culprit—infection (like COVID-19), disorder, injury, or toxin—has left. It is a health problem and has been linked to prolonged stress and autoimmune disorders (diseases that cause the body to attack itself). As a chronic issue, the inflammation progresses slowly, most often without our awareness. Chronic inflammation can progress to a host of other chronic disorders, affecting health and longevity. Some of these disorders are cardiovascular disease, cancer, diabetes, and arthritis. We'll learn about some food sources that are effective for combatting systemic inflammation in later chapters.

Risk factors associated with chronic inflammation include age, obesity, diet, smoking, low sex hormones, sleep disorders, infection, and stress. We cannot do anything about aging, but we can quit smoking and age more healthily by focusing on diet and exercise. Common signs (objective measurements) and symptoms (subjective measurements) of chronic inflammation include body pain, fatigue, insomnia, depression, moodiness, constipation, diarrhea, acid reflux, frequent infections, and weight gain. Phew! That was quite a list. Many of these signs and symptoms are common to other disorders not necessarily linked to inflammation. However, one biomarker of inflammation found in blood plasma is C-reactive protein. Circulating levels of this protein rise in response to inflammation. Another indicator of inflammation is something called a cytokine. Cytokines are small proteins involved with the immune response, so they are important in health and disease, specifically trauma, cancer, and inflammation. Blood tests can measure the concentration of C-reactive protein and pro-inflammatory cytokines and provide us with clues about our inflammation status.

Dietary measures aimed at reducing or removing inflammation triggers—those substances that set off the inflammatory response—include following a low-glycemic diet; reducing saturated fat and trans-fat; and eating plenty of fruits, vegetables, high-fiber foods, and nuts. Behavioral measures include exercising regularly, sleeping longer, and stressing less. This book will focus on nutritional measures and behavioral changes for optimizing health and well-being.

Food Allergy

We spent a lot of time talking about inflammation because it oftentimes is at the root of many health issues. Keep inflammation in check and we're off to a good start in battling disease. Yet, what we eat can *cause* an immune reaction. Inflammation and the immune reaction go hand-in-hand. When we speak of immune reactions, we are talking about the way our body responds to a specific substance.

With allergies, the body is responding to a particular allergen, which is usually a protein. Common allergies are to pollen, dust, and fur, but we can also be allergic to particular proteins in food. In each case, regardless of whether the allergy is environmental or part of the food we eat, the body is hypersensitive to the little protein. Not everybody has allergies, and allergies are as individual as any person is.

When an allergy arises, the immune system responds by releasing histamine, a chemical that causes inflammation. If the body cannot overcome the allergy, anaphylactic shock occurs. Anaphylactic shock is a serious, life-threatening condition in which the whole body responds with shortness of breath, low blood pressure, itchy rash, and throat and tongue swelling. Epinephrine is given to counteract the shock by opening airways, maintaining heartbeat, and restoring blood pressure.

A food allergy is an abnormal immune response to food. Common foods to which people are allergic include cow's milk, eggs, peanuts, tree nuts, and shellfish. Food allergies affect 5 percent of adults and 8 percent of children. Genetics and lifestyle may play a role in food allergy development. Management of food allergies includes avoidance of the specific culprit and preparedness—not always an easy task. And the first event of an immune reaction is inflammation.

But there are two main types of immune reactions to food, namely (1) food sensitivity/food intolerance and (2) food allergy. To be clear, a food allergy is not the same as a food sensitivity/intolerance. When a food allergy exists, like a person is allergic to shellfish, the body mounts an immune response to the food. The immune response is working to protect you from what the body perceives as a foreign protein. In this example, the foreign protein is something in the shellfish. That something is likely tropomyosin (TM), as more than 60 percent of people with shellfish allergies react to TM. Food allergies with subsequent immune responses are dangerous, leading to systemic reactions that can be life threatening.

Newer treatments and recommendations for food allergies are aimed at exposing children to the specific allergy in incremental amounts over time to desensitize them to the allergen. Studies are currently underway to test antibody injections as a therapy for peanut allergy. The antibodies neutralize the allergen, and pilot studies are showing promise. One such pilot study showed that an antibody injection stops peanut allergy for two to six weeks. More research is on the horizon, so stay tuned.

Contrast a food allergy with food sensitivity, which is another term for food intolerance. Food sensitivity/intolerance does not cause a full-blown reaction. It is generally just something quite uncomfortable. For example, with lactose intolerance, which is a reaction to the milk sugar lactose, the body has difficulty digesting the food. This can lead to bloating, gas, and belly aches. Once the lactose is eliminated, the person will be fine. It is not a life-threating situation.

When it comes to hoaxes centered around identifying food allergies, there is no shortage. There's a bit of hokum making the circuit now, and it relates to food allergies and the IgG test. First of all, IgG is the abbreviation for immunoglobulin G, which is a type of antibody. We have several immunoglobulin antibodies, and they are cleverly named IgM, IgA, IgD, IgG, and IgE. If you're paying close attention, you'll notice that the various types spell the name *MADGE*. Each letter stands for a different type of globulin (protein): macro (M), alpha (A), delta (D), and gamma (G). E is an outlier and was named after fraction E for inducing erythema (skin redness).

This particular antibody, IgG, is the most common type of antibody circulating in our blood and plays a major role in immunity. One way antibodies work is to bind to specific disease-causing organisms (pathogens), such as viruses and bacteria, and render them harmless. This binding works well to protect us from infection.

Measuring the level of IgG in the blood is an excellent tool for diagnosing certain conditions. When IgG levels are elevated, it is indicative of infection—elevated levels indicate your body is working to keep the infection at bay—or it indicates immunity to a particular agent. For example, if you aren't sure if you had a particular vaccine as a child, and you want to know if you are immune to a particular infectious agent, your blood can be checked for the antibody to that agent.

Testing IgG levels is not indicative of allergy. Thus, the IgG food panel test marketed by various companies that claims to diagnose food sensitivities is not supported by science. It reports IgG levels to various foods and claims that removing foods with high IgG levels will improve symptoms. The Internet is rich with stories and unfounded reports claiming the test will enable you to tweak your diet and subsequently ease symptoms of autism, cystic fibrosis, epilepsy, irritable bowel syndrome, and rheumatoid arthritis. Elevated levels of IgG may simply be due to the presence of food and likely *tolerance*—not *intolerance*—to those foods. This test is not supported by medical professionals. The American Academy of Allergy, Asthma & Immunology, the Canadian Society of Allergy and Clinical Immunology, and the European Academy of Allergy and Clinical Immunology have all advised against using this test to diagnose food intolerance/food sensitivity.

Colon Cleansing

Colon cleansing, also called a colonic or colonic irrigation, falls into the category of gastrointestinal quackery. It's quackery because the job of the colon is already to rid the body of wastes. There is one area in which colon cleansing does serve a purpose: before medical procedures like a colonoscopy, evacuating the bowels is a good thing. In preparation for such a procedure, one usually drinks copious amounts of fluids with a laxative to get the intestines squeaky clean.

In other cases, voluminous amounts of water and possibly coffee and herbs, are flushed through the colon using a tube inserted into the rectum. This should be avoided. Risks include dehydration, bowel perforation, infection, electrolyte imbalance, kidney failure, and possibly death. The risks of colonic cleansing certainly outweigh any perceived benefits.

Microbiome, Prebiotics and Probiotics

It seems that any time the digestive system is discussed, the conversation turns to the microbiome. What is this microbiome? The microorganisms, or microbes for short, living within the intestines are referred to as the gut microbiome, intestinal flora, microflora or micro-biota—to name a few. All terms mean the same. While we have millions of microbes living *on* us, we'll focus on those living *in* us, with the vast majority residing in the intestines. Information regarding the link between these microscopic residents and human disease is expanding. For example, scientists are discovering that the gut microbiome in people with inflammatory bowel disease is different from the gut flora of healthy people.

Once again, we have to turn to our human history as we have evolved with microbes over millennia. We generally think of microbes as being harmful and something we should eradiate, but the truth is that we need them—as long as they are the right type and in the right place. What are bacteria good for? They digest fiber, affect gut health, produce vitamins, may reduce cholesterol, and function in immunity.

The relationship we have with the gut microbiome is mutualistic, meaning it is beneficial to us and them. To illustrate, bacteria in the gut ferment dietary fiber into short-chain fatty acids. This also produces gas and is the reason you have flatulence after eating beans. Intestinal bacteria also synthesize B complex vitamins (important for cellular metabolism) and vitamin K (important to blood clotting). The resident bacteria also keep harmful bacteria in check. Dysregulation of the microbiome is correlated with inflammation and autoimmune disorders. A 2018 study in *Behavioural Brain Research* found that acute and repeated exposure to social stress reduced the gut microbiome in hamsters. Further research is needed to determine if this occurs in humans but recall the association between *Helicobacter pylori* and stomach ulcers.

Development of the gut microbiome takes time, but the gut microbiome of infants is established through the birth process itself (coming in contact with vaginal microbes), being around other people (community microbes), breast milk, and food. Caesarean section (C-section) and formula feeding affect the composition of the intestinal microflora.

Recent studies have also found that the microbiota of vaginally-delivered babies is different from babies born by C-section. C-section babies lacked strains of commensal bacteria, which are typically found in vaginally-delivered babies. With commensal bacteria, different strains live harmoniously with one deriving benefit and the other deriving neither benefit nor harm. The guts of babies born by C-section were dominated with *Enterococcus* and *Klebsiella* bacteria, which are opportunistic. Opportunistic microorganisms cause infection in patients with depressed immune systems, meaning that healthy people can typically prevent opportunists from taking over. The health effect of these findings is currently under study. Epidemiological research has suggested that babies born by C-section are at increased risk of developing asthma and obesity. Swabbing one's vagina and inoculating C-section newborns has been done by well-meaning parents, but medical professionals advise against the practice.

Probiotics and prebiotics are a relatively hot area of research right now. Daily science and non-science newsfeeds often have an article about each. But what are they? Probiotics are foods you eat that contain live bacteria and yeasts. Yogurt, fresh sauerkraut, and fermented foods are probiotics. Prebiotics are high-fiber foods such as fruits, vegetables, and whole grains that feed the bacteria in your gut. Think of them as fertilizer for what's already there. Both support helpful gut bacteria. If you are "on the go" and want to consume some probiotics, grab a yogurt, which contains the most common probiotic, *Lactobacillus*. If you want to consume some prebiotics, grab some type of high-fiber food.

Much is yet to be learned about *how* they work, but we do know that it's important to consume them during and after a course of antibiotics. Antibiotics can kill off the good bacteria in your gut, so the probiotics can help replace them. They also can help keep bacteria in your gut in balance. An entire book could be written on this topic, especially as more is known about the benefits of bacteria.

Understanding the nutritional role of both prebiotics and probiotics is in its infancy. Despite it being a young field, probiotic supplements were a $35 billion enterprise in 2015; sales are projected to exceed $65 billion by 2024. Since probiotic pills are supplements and not food, they are not regulated by the FDA, and therefore may not contain the ingredients or amounts listed on the label. If a pill bottle carries the USP (U.S. Pharmacopeia Convention) label, the contents should be as described. It cannot be stressed enough: we should eat the actual food versus taking a supplement whenever possible.

3

It's a Whale of a Time
Weight Control and Calories

Weight Control

When it comes to weight control, there is no magic bullet. What we do have is nutrition, exercise, and therapy. Bookshelves and websites are quite literally stuffed with information and misinformation about the best way to control weight. It's astonishing really, because a varied, balanced diet in conjunction with physical activity are all we generally need to stay healthy. I write "generally" because many times there are underlying psychological and environmental issues that should be considered. Emerging research has shown that many factors contribute to weight and body mass index (BMI) including posttraumatic stress; childhood/adolescent physical, emotional, and sexual abuse; depression; intimate partner violence; incest; and other sociological events. Taken together or separately, each increases the risk for overweight and obesity and contributes to overweight prevalence and difficulty in maintaining a healthy body weight. In cases of abuse, eating may be the only way individuals can exert any control over their lives. The weight becomes a shield.

Goals of this book are to give you science-based information so that you can make sensible choices about how you live. This chapter focuses on weight control and calories. A good place to start is by explaining the different ways our body burns calories.

First up is basal metabolic rate. The term *basal* means base or bottom, and the basal metabolic rate (BMR) is the same thing as resting metabolic rate (RMR). Physiologically, the BMR/RMR is the number of calories we burn just through our body systems functioning. Think heart beating, muscles contracting, simple breathing, and sleeping. The BMR depends on a number of factors, including age, weight, and sex, but the majority of our calories are spent just keeping us alive. You can find online calculators to determine yours, but here is a general formula:

> Females: resting metabolic rate = 655 + (4.35 × weight in pounds) + (4.7 × height in inches) − (4.7 × age in years)
>
> Males: resting metabolic rate = 66 + (6.23 × weight in pounds) + (12.7 × height in inches) − (6.8 × age in years)

Example: Female, 115 pounds, 60 inches, 54 years

655 + (4.35 × 115) + (4.7 × 60) − (4.7 × 54)

655 + (500.25) + (282) − (253.8)

1,183.45 ~ 1,183 calories

The second way calories are burned is the thermic effect of food (TEF). These are the calories we burn through digestion. Recall from the previous chapter that the mere act of digesting our food burns calories. This value can vary greatly depending on the proportions of proteins, carbohydrates, and fats in your diet. Here is the breakdown:

- Proteins take the most energy to digest—20–30 percent of total protein calories eaten go toward digesting protein
- Carbohydrates are next—5–10 percent of total carbohydrate calories eaten go toward digesting carbohydrate
- Fats are last—0–3 percent of total fat calories eaten go toward digesting fat

At one time, people believed that some foods might have a negative calorie effect. For example, you might think that it takes more calories to digest celery than you actually derive from that stalk of celery. But that's not true. There are no foods that burn more calories than they contain.

The third way we burn calories is through exercise, the so-called exercise-related activity thermogenesis (EAT). This is the deliberate type of exercise that involves heading to the gym, lifting weights, riding a bicycle, playing sports, and the like. Interestingly, this type of exercise accounts for very little of our calorie burning. Again, there is individual variation and if you are a professional athlete, say a basketball player or Olympic sprinter, then disregard the non-calorie burning effect of exercise-related thermogenesis. For the rest of us, diet—what we put into our mouths—is going to play a bigger role in weight loss than does exercise.

The fourth way we burn calories is through non-exercise thermogenesis (NEAT). This is different than BMR. These are the calories spent in activities of daily living, such as going to work, walking to and from your car, and the like. NEAT calories are highly variable and individual behaviors can significantly affect daily energy expenditure. Research has shown that a low level of NEAT is associated with obesity.

Let's get back to the role of diet. Diet refers to the food you eat regularly, not some particular, specially-named diet. Diet is the healthy food you want to consume day in and day out for the rest of your life. It's what keeps you at lower risk for future diseases, and we know moderation is key. This doesn't mean eating way less all the time, it means eating the appropriate foods in the right amounts. If you were to suddenly start eating less food, you might find that initially you don't lose any weight. This is because your metabolism slows down, too. There's nothing you can do about this—except really exercise—because your body is evolutionarily programmed to conserve for those periods of famine. So what you need to do is figure out how to eat well to stay well.

Fat and Obesity

Under a microscope, fat looks like water droplets in flattened Jell-O. However, it is not water but metabolically active adipose tissue. You can appreciate how fat is a tissue if you've ever seen greasy fat strips surrounding a hunk of meat. First identified in 1551 by Swiss naturalist Conrad Gessner, we now know that fat is also recognized as an endocrine organ because it produces hormones. Those hormones include leptin, estrogen, resistin, and cytokine. It's also interesting to note that we have two types of fat, white adipose tissue (WAT) and brown adipose tissue (BAT), and each has particular functions. White adipose tissue stores energy and brown adipose tissue generates body heat. Curiously, the exact physiology of the adipose tissue can vary depending on where it is located, and fat deposits vary between the sexes. Furthermore, the proportions change throughout life and the formation of fat tissue is likely controlled by an adipose gene.

Just as there are health risks to being underweight, there are problems with being overweight. We generally refer to being overweight as being fat. However, for optimal health, fat is necessary. Fat is needed to make hormones, provide thermal insulation, serve as a shock absorber, and store energy for use when necessary. Accumulating too much is not healthy, though, and too much weight is associated with increased disease risk. Accordingly, fat distribution is more critical than "over fatness"—a topic we'll discuss next.

So how much is too much body fat? It depends on the person and being fat is different than being obese. By health definition, obesity is excessively high body fat in relation to lean body tissue (muscle). Some terms associated with obesity and fatness are central obesity and intra-abdominal fat. Central obesity refers to excess fat found in the abdomen and around the body trunk, the "central" part of the whole body. This is "belly fat" and looks like the proverbial beer gut. No six-pack abs but rather kegger abs. Intra-abdominal fat is excess fat that is stored within the abdominal cavity and is associated with fat attached directly to abdominal organs. These abdominal organs are known as *viscera*, so this type of fat is called *visceral fat*. Any time you see the term *viscera*, automatically think *organ*. When visceral fat surrounds the heart, it is called *epicardial fat*, derived from the term *epi* meaning *around* and *cardial* meaning *heart*. While a little is okay because fat cushions organs, too much visceral fat leads to diseases like diabetes, stroke, hypertension, and decreased mortality (shorter life). Subcutaneous fat is non-visceral fat that is found just under the skin's surface, between the skin and underlying organs.

Unlike visceral fat and epicardial fat, subcutaneous fat is generally not associated with disease. Let that sink in for a moment as we consider Sumo wrestlers, who eat up to 7,000 calories each day and weigh 300–400 pounds. The Japanese word *sumo* means "striking one another" and the goal of the full contact sport is to force the opponent out of the circle. These grapplers are very strong, but outward appearance suggests they must be unhealthy. Yet, CT scans show that Sumo wrestlers don't have much visceral fat at all. The majority of their fat is subcutaneous fat, stored just below the skin's surface, and for this reason, they are considered healthy.

Although there are numerous ways to measure your fat, one simple test to determine health risk is to measure your waist-to-hip ratio (WHR). The World Health Organization states that having a waist-to-hip ratio over 1.0 increases the risk of developing heart disease and type 2 diabetes. In fact, the WHR may be a better measure of risk, even if a person's body mass index (weight-to-height ratio) is within normal range. Body mass index (BMI) is discussed shortly. Here's the WHR formula for measuring your risk of disease.

Relative Risk for Disease Formula

1. measure your waist circumference
2. measure your hip circumference
3. divide waist circumference number by hip circumference number
   Ratio of .80 or more in females = risk
   Ratio of .95 or more in males = risk

Here's an example:

Sex: Female
Waist circumference: 26 inches
Hip circumference: 36 inches
Calculation: 26/36 = .72, low health risk

See the chart below for relative risk for disease for females and males using WHR.

Health Risk for Females and Males Using Waist-to-Hip Ratio

Health Risk	Females	Males
Low	0.80 or lower	0.95 or lower
Moderate	0.81–0.85	0.96–1.0
High	0.86 or higher	1.1 or higher

Just as there is no perfect formula for all people, causes of obesity are interrelated, meaning there is no one particular cause. What we do know is that we're all different. One unproven and controversial theory that still makes headlines is the set-point theory. The word "theory" here is not the scientific use but rather the common vernacular use which means supposition. It's an idea to explain something. This theory states that the body maintains a certain weight by means of its own internal controls. Proponents of this idea cite some twin studies showing that heredity determines weight and that there is a genetic tendency to store fat, even when intakes are comparable. Similar to the set-point theory is "anatomic predetermination," which proposes that anatomic features, including fat deposition, are genetically destined for their location as well as the timing of their appearance on the body. In essence, if you want to know where your fat will deposit 20 years from now, take a look at your mom.

Behavior also plays a role. Fat is highly palatable, so we like to indulge and over-indulge. It has been suggested that we have a primitive fear of starvation, so we eat, even in times of feast when famine likely won't happen. And sometimes we're overweight because we simply expend too little energy.

Weight Control and Calories

An important nutritional concept in weight control is caloric need. The scientific definition of a calorie is the energy needed to raise the temperature of one gram of water 1°C. For our purposes, we'll define calories as food energy. One gram of carbohydrates has four calories, one gram of fat has nine calories, and one gram of protein has four calories. One pound of body weight is approximately 3,500 calories. Recall that your body has a preferential use of energy and will use the energy from carbohydrates first, followed by fats, and then proteins. At rest, fat makes up about 85 percent of our calories burned. As you exercise, the percentage shifts: if you start walking, about 70 percent of calories burned are fat calories, and if you increase to a moderate run, the mix becomes 50 percent fat and 50 percent carbohydrates, and if you start running full on, calories burned shifts toward more carbohydrates being used for fuel. If your goal is to burn fat, a check you can use is the "talking while running test"—if you can talk while you run, you're burning some fat; if you can't talk while running, your body shifts to carbohydrate metabolism.

If you are curious about your own daily calorie requirements, you can figure it out yourself. To determine the approximate number of calories you need every day, first determine your body weight and then choose one of the following formulas:

- Weight Maintenance: multiply body weight ×
  15 calories/pound
- Weight Reduction: multiply body weight ×
  10 calories/pound
- Weight Gain: multiply body weight × 20 calories/pound

Here's an example: If you weigh 115 pounds and want to maintain your current weight at your current activity level multiple 115 by 15 to get 1,725 calories.

Basal Metabolic Rate (BMR), Body Mass Index (BMI) and Healthy Weight

Time to turn our attention to basal metabolic rate and body mass index. The number of calories you need to consume to maintain basic body functions such as breathing and keeping your heart beating is known as the *basal metabolic rate* (BMR). The BMR is an estimate of how many calories you burn doing nothing but resting—it does not include daily activities or exercise. Physiologists use equations to figure this out, but online calculators using the Mifflin-St. Jeor equation are pretty good sources to try if you want to calculate your BMR. These calculators require the following information: current weight, height, age, and sex. For a five-foot, 50-year-old woman who weighs 115 pounds, the estimated BMR is 1,063 calories per day. Compare this figure with the one above for maintaining body weight. The difference is 662 calories, showing that just "existing" burns calories! Tweaking that calculator and adding 30 years, this same 5-foot woman will only need 913 calories per day when she is 80. A five-foot, 115-pound, 50-year-old male needs 1,219 calories, but when he is 80, he'll need 1,069 calories. You can see how caloric intake varies by age and sex.

Another calculation used to estimate your ideal weight is using the body mass index (BMI). This value is calculated from a person's weight (in kilograms—kg) and height (in meters—m and centimeters—cm). It provides a somewhat reliable (more about that statement) late indicator of body fatness for most people and is used to screen for weight categories that may lead to health problems. That said, there are still clinical limitations because BMI is a measure of excess weight, not excess fat—that means that BMI does not directly measure body fat. Recall the case of our Sumo wrestlers, who by BMI measures would be considered prime candidates for health risks. Many factors, such as age, sex, and muscle mass, influence BMI values. Therefore, some people, such as athletes and weightlifters, may have a BMI that identifies them as overweight even though they do not have excess body fat. Or as is often the case, a few extra pounds get added on because in many instances, body weight and height are measured in your doctor's office where you walk in, stand on the scales fully dressed, and your weight and height are measured. These numbers are plugged into a formula and voila, the BMI is calculated. Like the athlete example, the value may not be totally accurate. The take-home message here is that BMI is an imperfect tool and its impact on some disease risks and outcomes are not assured.

There are many online calculators you can use to identify your BMI. But if you'd like to exercise your brain and do it by hand, here is the formula and an example for a person who is five feet (60 inches) tall and weighs 120 pounds:

STEP 1: Multiply the weight in pounds (lbs.) by 0.45 (the metric conversion factor) to get kilograms (kg)

120 lbs. × 0.45 = 54 kg

STEP 2: Multiply the height in inches by 0.025 (the metric conversion factor) to get meters (m)

60 in. × 0.025 = 1.5 meters (m)

STEP 3: Square the answer from step 2 above

1.5 m × 1.5 m = 2.25 m

STEP 4: Divide the answer from step 1 above by the answer from step 3

54 kg/2.25 m = 24, the BMI for a person who is 5 feet tall and weighs 120 pounds.

Knowing your BMI can be revealing, because maintaining a healthy weight reduces the risk of certain diseases. Using the BMI chart from the Centers for Disease Control and Prevention (CDC) (below), we see this person has a healthy weight. Go ahead and calculate your own BMI and see where you fall.

Body Mass Index (BMI) Table

BMI	*Considered*
Below 18.5	Underweight
18.5 to 24.9	Healthy weight
25.0 to 29.9	Overweight
30 or higher	Obese

A few paragraphs back I mentioned that BMI is a "somewhat reliable indicator." The reason I used inexact language is because BMI was never intended to be used in the manner in which we use it today. Its inventor was Adolphe Quetelet, a 19th-century academic with varied interests in studying astronomy, mathematics, statistics, and sociology, but not medicine. His intention was to serve as a statistical measurement of populations, not individuals. In so doing, individual health could not be measured. But what was measured was the size and measurements of French and Scottish white men, basically Western Europeans. The scale was called Quetelet's Index and was used as scientific justification for eugenics. This index made its way into 20th-century life when U.S. life insurance companies compiled height and weight tables for actuarial purposes.

It wasn't until the 1970s that another set of researchers was looking for an easy measure of fatness that could be used in a medical setting. Like their predecessors, this group, led by researcher Ancel Keys, assessed men of predominantly white countries (United States, Finland, and Italy) plus Japan and South Africa. There is a caveat to studying South African men: the findings applied to South African men except for Bantu men. The name was changed from Quetelet's Index to Body Mass Index and studies found it to be accurate in diagnosing obesity about 50 percent of the time.

Fast forward to 2011 when an article in *Journal of Obstetrics and Gynecology* found BMI to be a poor indicator of fatness. In fact, BMI was not accurate in detecting obesity in various female populations. This makes sense since the studies were never done using women or a cross section of people.

In 2015, researchers at Harvard University and the University of Sheffield identified six different types of obese person:

1. Young healthy females
2. Heavy-drinking males
3. Unhappy and anxious middle-aged
4. Affluent and healthy older-aged
5. Physically sick but happy older-aged
6. Poorest health

By 2016, researchers at Massachusetts General Hospital identified 59 different types of obesity. Yet, BMI still remains at the forefront as the measure for determining health risks—despite its flaws. From a scientific perspective, determining fitness, fatness, healthiness, and health risk is a complex science.

What is certain is that for optimum health, one needs a balanced diet. Such a diet contains an adequate daily amount of carbohydrates, fats, proteins, vitamins, minerals, and water. Basic nutritional status is determined by evaluating the person's weight, height, energy level, 24-hour dietary recall, history of weight loss/gain, and specific dietary patterns or beliefs. If more in-depth nutritional assessment is necessary, health professionals will conduct an evaluation that includes laboratory tests, physical examination, and dietary analysis. However, if you are eating well, getting enough exercise, and maintaining the weight you want, then that's generally all you need.

Worldwide, 11.3 percent of the population is hungry. That number represents about 805 million people who eat less than the recommended 2,100 calories per day. Yet, the diet industry thrives because obesity has reached pandemic proportions, and Americans' need for quick fixes have reached epidemic proportions. According to the CDC, the prevalence of obesity and being overweight is staggeringly high. Their statistics show the following: 35.9 percent of adults aged 20 and over are obese and 69.2 percent of U.S. adults 20 years and over are overweight, including being obese. It doesn't help the average person to understand the difference between "obese" and "overweight" because the criteria center on *ranges*. To illustrate, the CDC provides the following definition:

> Overweight and obesity are both labels for ranges of weight that are greater than what is generally considered healthy for a given height. The terms also identify ranges of weight that have been shown to increase the likelihood of certain diseases and other health problems. For adults, overweight and obesity ranges are determined by using weight and height to calculate a number called the "body mass index" (BMI). BMI is used because, for most people, it correlates with their amount of body fat.
>
> - An adult who has a BMI between 25 and 29.9 is considered overweight.
> - An adult who has a BMI of 30 or higher is considered obese.

That's a lot to take in when the simple definition of obesity is having too much fat. And we all probably know when we have too much fat.

Obesity occurs as a result of many factors, such as sedentary lifestyle, eating too much, not getting enough rest, genetic factors, and some medications. We also know that childhood eating patterns such as snacking could be a contributor to childhood obesity. Long-term obesity is associated with serious medical conditions including type 2 diabetes mellitus, hypertension (high blood pressure), some cancers, sleep apnea, and heart disease. We know that losing weight can reduce and/or reverse these conditions.

Strategies for Weight Loss

A strategy for weight loss is to cut calories and increase activity levels. As a refresher, one pound of body fat equals 3500 calories. To lose a pound per week, you'd have to cut 500 calories per day. A realistic eating plan is in order, though. The average person—whoever that person is—needs at least 15 calories per pound to maintain their weight.

Losing weight can be hard and a problem with repeated dieting is that this creates weight cycling whereby cycles of weight loss are offset by subsequent weight gains, usually to a higher weight. This is known as the yo-yo effect or the ratchet effect. For this reason, the ideal weight control plan centers on eating sensibly and exercising regularly. This is always better than any "dieting."

Bariatric Surgery

Important to bring up at this point is the use of bariatric surgery for weight loss. Bariatrics is the branch of medicine dealing with the prevention and control of obesity and its associated diseases. There are several types of bariatric surgeries—namely gastric band, gastric sleeve, gastric bypass, and duodenal switch—and each type has its own advantages and disadvantages. Each causes weight loss, but the mechanism varies from restricting the amount of food that the stomach can hold, to causing malabsorption of nutrients, or to a combination of restriction and malabsorption. Evidence shows that bariatric surgical treatments result in greater weight loss than nonsurgical treatments. Five-year follow-up studies have shown weight loss, less diabetes, and blood lipid improvements. However, more information is needed about long-term outcomes, complications following the procedures, long-term survival, vascular events, mental health outcomes, and cost.

Additionally, when the stomach or portions of the stomach are removed, people face vitamin B12 deficiency because of a loss of the chemical called intrinsic factor. Intrinsic factor is produced by parietal cells in the stomach and its role is to bind vitamin B12 for absorption in the small intestine. If the cells are no longer there because the stomach is no longer there, then there will be no intrinsic factor. For this reason, lifelong dietary vitamin B12 supplementation is necessary. Vitamin B12, discussed in Chapter 7, is also needed to make red blood cells. Without adequate red blood cell formation, people become anemic.

Anorexia Nervosa, Bulimia Nervosa and Binge-Eating Disorder

Eating disorders are not lifestyle choices. In fact, eating disorders are serious fatal illnesses characterized by disturbances in eating behaviors with preoccupation with food, body weight, and shape. Before getting into the differences between anorexia nervosa and bulimia nervosa, the term *anorexia* must be defined. Anorexia is derived from the word parts *an* meaning *without* and *orexis* meaning *appetite*. Although it is commonplace for the terms anorexia and anorexia nervosa to be used interchangeably, they are not the same condition. Anorexia is an umbrella term that means a diminished appetite or an aversion to food. Appetite, a natural, psychological desire for food, is different than hunger, which is a feeling of discomfort caused by lack of food. One can precede the other. When you are sick and don't feel like eating, you have anorexia. Hospital patients who are too sick to eat have anorexia. When you look at or smell food and it appeals to you, you have an appetite.

Anorexia occurs with a chronic illness that makes food unpalatable, so you do not eat because you just are not hungry. This is not a hunger strike or a fast. A person who is fasting chooses not to eat. Fasting people abstain from all or some kinds of food or beverages. Mahatma Gandhi (1869–1948), Father of the Nation of India, was an Indian nationalist and spiritual leader who fasted at different times during India's freedom movement. The practice of fasting has a long history dating back thousands of years. Sometimes fasting is done in protest or civil disobedience; sometimes it is done for religious reasons, and sometimes it is done in preparation for medical tests. Regardless, the purposes are varied. Intermittent fasting, eating every other day, eating five days per week, or just cutting back every other day, may have health benefits such as weight loss and less inflammation, a topic further explored in Chapter 9.

Anorexia nervosa is a medical and psychological disorder that manifests as an extreme fear of becoming overweight and is accompanied by food aversion. Anorexia nervosa is a compulsive pursuit of thinness at the expense of good health. People with anorexia nervosa see themselves as being overweight, regardless of how much they weigh. Much has been written about this disorder, which is characterized by steady weight loss to and below 85 percent of normal weight for height. Individuals with anorexia nervosa achieve profound weight loss through not eating, strenuous exercise, self-induced vomiting to rid the body of recently-eaten food, and laxatives to rid the body of excess water and feces.

From a physiological standpoint, there is profound muscle wasting—a condition called *muscle atrophy*. The subcutaneous fat just below the skin's surface diminishes to the point where there is very little to none. This is followed by a slew of other conditions such as anemia (not enough iron in the blood), electrolyte (mineral) imbalance, bradycardia (slow heart rate), hypotension (low blood pressure), asthenia (abnormal physical weakness and lack of energy), exaggerated cold sensitivity, constipation, dry skin with increased pigmentation, and growth of lanugo (fine, soft hair). Women become amenorrheal (failure to menstruate). The risk of osteoporosis (a loss of bone density leading to brittleness), fractures, and irreversible bone deformation increases due to lack of minerals such as calcium and phosphorus, and also due to hormonal imbalance. In short, it is a life-threatening eating disorder and is marked by extreme weight loss. If treated in its early stages, anorexia nervosa can be reversed; treatment in later stages is typically not successful. In 1983, American musician Karen Carpenter died at age 32 as a result of anorexia nervosa.

People with bulimia nervosa, oftentimes referred to just as bulimia, eat large volumes of food at frequent intervals. They feel a lack of control over this over-eating and then compensate by trying to rid the body of the food. Ways of getting rid of the food include forced vomiting, using laxatives or diuretics, excessively exercising, and fasting. People with bulimia nervosa can be underweight, normal weight, or overweight.

Symptoms of bulimia nervosa include chronic sore throat and worn tooth enamel due to persistent exposure to the acidic stomach contents flushing the throat and coating the teeth from vomiting. Dehydration and subsequent electrolyte imbalance occur as a result of purging fluids through laxative and diuretic use. Electrolyte imbalance, particularly of sodium, calcium, and potassium, can lead to heart attack, stroke, and death.

Binge-eating disorder is characterized by a person's inability to control their eating. People with binge-eating disorder eat too much, too often. Unlike anorexia nervosa and bulimia nervosa, eating is not followed by any sort of purging. It is the most common eating disorder in the United States and leads to being overweight or obese.

Treatments and therapies for all eating disorders aim to alleviate the psychological issue first. Thus, psychotherapy, oftentimes coupled with medication, is appropriate. Nutritional counseling is necessary while medical care and monitoring is needed.

Cachexia

Contrast eating disorders with cachexia, which is a wasting syndrome marked by overall ill health, weight loss, and muscle loss. The word *cachexia* comes from the Greek word *kakos* that means *bad* plus the suffix -*hexis*, which means *condition of the body*. On the outside, cachexia looks like anorexia nervosa; the difference is that the weight loss and muscle wasting occur as a result of a chronic disease, like cancer or AIDS. To help you remember this word, think about the abbreviation for cancer, which is CA. The letters C and A are the first two letters of the word *cachexia*.

Treatment is complex because the underlying disease must be treated or in remission. People with cachexia generally respond poorly to treatment, which is aimed at the wasting syndrome itself; they also have a very short survival time and suffer greatly. They have no energy, are extremely tired, are chronically fatigued with very little exertion, and have a very low quality of life. It's a horrible condition because the person no longer likes the way they look; they have difficulty interacting with other people, including their own family; eating is very troublesome; and social interactions become increasingly difficult. While writing this book, I had a front-row seat to the ravages of cancer and its concomitant cachexia: Within nine months of diagnosis for kidney cancer, my 205-pound brother lost 105 pounds and died. Before his death, he looked like a skeleton with skin covering his bones. He looked like a walking dead man would look—if only he were able to walk. He could barely walk because he had so little energy. Although cancer drugs (chemotherapy) were beating back the cancer, his cachexia was so far advanced that nothing could save him.

Cachexia has such an effect on a person that studies of people in palliative care settings showed that cachexia was within the top five most troubling symptom cluster. It ranked above pain and difficulty breathing. Diagnostic criteria for cachexia exist; however, once you've seen it, you know it. In a medical setting, basic criteria include a five-pound weight loss in the preceding two months without trying to lose weight or an estimated caloric intake of less than 20 calories per kilogram (2.2 pounds) of body weight.

Putting that into perspective, a 220-pound person weighs 100 kilograms. Twenty calories times 100 kilograms = 2,000 calories. Nutritional counseling and eating more food have relatively little to no effect. People with cachexia simply don't feel like eating, and if they *are* able to eat, the body cannot utilize the calories in a normal fashion.

When comparing cachexia with anorexia, it is important to realize that cachexia is a complex pathophysiological metabolic syndrome and anorexia is a nutritional deficiency. Simply put: You can treat anorexia by eating; but eating cannot treat cachexia. In fact, once cachexia has reached a critical point, it cannot even be reversed, despite any type of nutrition or drug therapy. The tissue wasting and multiple organ system involvement is just too profound.

When considering what is best for you, your personal goals should be front and center, keeping in mind what you've just learned about caloric intake and caloric need relative to health. In the upcoming chapters, we'll explore the role of macronutrients and micronutrients in our diets.

4

How Sweet It Is

Carbohydrates—Sugar,
Glycogen and Fiber

Dietary Carbohydrates

Carbohydrates 101 begins with the very straightforward point that we need carbohydrates to fuel our body cells. But what are carbohydrates? Put simply, carbohydrates are macronutrients including various sugars, starch, glycogen, and fiber and are found in fruits, vegetables, milk, grains, seeds, nuts, and legumes. While nuts and legumes are generally classified as proteins, nuts and legumes do have a little carbohydrate (starch) and fiber. All carbohydrates contain four calories per gram of carbohydrate. The Dietary Guidelines for Americans recommends that carbohydrates make up 45 percent–65 percent of your total daily calories with less than 10 percent coming from added sugars. For a typical 2,000 calories per day diet, 900–1,300 calories (225–325 grams) should be from carbohydrates. No worries about getting enough: Americans get plenty of carbohydrates from sugar and related sweeteners, consuming about 77 pounds per person per year of the sweet stuff. Grab a piece of candy and read on.

As a class, carbohydrates are organic compounds found in food and living tissues—animals and plants. Organic means that the compound contains carbon. From a chemical perspective, a carbohydrate molecule is abbreviated as CHO because it is made up of carbon (C), hydrogen (H), and oxygen (O) atoms. Carbon is the fourth most abundant element in the universe, following hydrogen, helium, and oxygen. We need carbohydrates and regardless of the type of carbohydrate, it will be broken down into simpler sugars to release energy in the form of ATP (more on this later). This means that no matter what, you need carbohydrates to generate ATP, which is the only source of energy that your body can use.

A common carbohydrate is glucose—a simple sugar. You probably have heard a person with diabetes say, "I've got sugar." *Sugar* refers to a specific type of sugar called *glucose*, and if a person has "sugar," they have diabetes. Most people with diabetes cannot metabolize or use glucose effectively without medication. Every cell in our body likes glucose, and these body cells are suspended within blood. We generally think of blood as a fluid, but we have to expand our understanding a bit. Blood is a circulating tissue, meaning that it is indeed a fluid, but other things, like cells and nutrients are suspended in it.

We discussed key structures of the digestive system in Chapter 2, but it helps to revisit them in context of their key functions. One such body structure is the pancreas, an organ that is crucial for carbohydrate/sugar/glucose metabolism. Situated within the first fold of the small intestine, it secretes two important hormones for regulating glucose: insulin and glucagon. These two hormones counteract each other to maintain glucose homeostasis. Insulin's job is to decrease blood glucose while glucagon's job is to increase blood glucose.

How the Body Uses Carbohydrates

Carbohydrates are used primarily for energy, and in the body, energy is in the form of a compound called adenosine triphosphate (ATP). ATP is to our body's functioning what gasoline is to your car's engine. In order to generate ATP, we need food, and that food needs to be broken down into a form the body *knows* what to do with it. If we did nothing but sit, we'd still need energy to maintain sitting, breathing, heart beating, and digesting—all those events that comprise our basal metabolism.

Now it's time to get a little sciency and discuss *how* we make ATP. Getting a basic understanding of this process is important so that you can debunk any diet fads on your own. Our innate biochemistry (how the major nutrients work in our bodies and why they are important) and thousands of years of evolution demand that we include carbohydrates, fats, proteins, vitamins, minerals, and water into our diets.

Within our body's cells, glucose is converted to ATP, our biochemical energy. Present in all living tissues, ATP fuels our cells. You are all familiar with cells running low on ATP: when you are out of energy, you get tired. Permanent shortage of ATP leads to death and manifests itself as rigor mortis. When you die, you no longer make ATP, muscles become stiff, and rigor mortis sets in. In fact, the term *rigor mortis* is derived from Latin and literally means "stiffness of death."

Before rigor occurs, we have a lifetime of glucose utilization. However, in order to be effective, that glucose has to get *into* our cells because it doesn't do any good out in the bloodstream. It can only do that by two ways: diffusion and insulin transport. Biologically, diffusion means that something in solution goes from a greater concentration to a lesser concentration. In your everyday life, diffusion occurs whenever you drop a sugar cube in your hot cup of tea: The sugar dissolves and disperses throughout the cup until uniformity is achieved.

Because glucose is so important to our big brains, brain cells obtain glucose by simple diffusion, in which glucose moves from the bloodstream into brain cells without an insulin transporter. In other body cells, insulin is necessary; otherwise, the glucose would remain in the bloodstream, causing blood levels to rise. People with diabetes mellitus oftentimes take injectable insulin to enable glucose to get from the bloodstream into their cells. The key point is that while our brains can obtain glucose by simple diffusion, other cells require insulin to transport glucose into the cell—kind of like hitching a ride.

Negative feedback mechanisms ensure glucose regulation. Recall from Chapter 2 that the hormone that works opposite insulin is glucagon, which ensures that the right amount of glucose remains in the bloodstream. It's a delicate physiological balancing act termed homeostasis. Homeostasis is achieved when the circulating level of blood glucose is maintained within a range of about 70–130 mg/dL, depending on the time of day and the time since a meal was eaten. The abbreviation "mg/dL" means *milligrams per deciliter*. The table below shows normal blood glucose ranges for a person *without* diabetes, according to the American Diabetes Association.

Normal Ranges for Blood Glucose

Times	Circulating Blood Glucose Level mg/dL
Fasting	Less than 100
1 hour after a meal	90–130
2 hours after a meal	90–110
5 or more hours after a meal	70–90

Hypoglycemia results if blood glucose is too low and *hyperglycemia* results if blood glucose is too high. These words are derived from the following word parts:

hypo- = low
hyper- = high
glyc = glucose, sugar
-emia = condition of the blood

Signs and symptoms of hypoglycemia include shakiness, weakness, clumsiness, difficulty talking, and confusion. Maintaining glucose balance is very important to feeding our cells; and if not treated, hypoglycemia can lead to loss of consciousness, seizures, and death.

Hyperglycemia is the opposite of hypoglycemia. A person may not be aware that they are hyperglycemic unless their blood glucose level is measured or if the hyperglycemic condition is extraordinarily high. Chronic (long-lasting) hyperglycemia can lead to serious complications such as cardiovascular disease, kidney disease, and damage to the retinas of the eyes.

Monitoring blood glucose at various times is important because it provides information on how well particular organs or hormones are working. The medical specialty concerned with hormone disorders like diabetes is endocrinology. Fasting hyperglycemia is defined as blood glucose above 130 mg/dL when you don't eat for at least eight hours. Postprandial hyperglycemia, also called *reactive hyperglycemia*, is defined as blood glucose above 180 mg/dL one to two hours after eating. The word *postprandial* means *after eating*, and results because the liver doesn't stop producing glucose as it normally would after eating a meal. While hyperglycemia is a common complication of diabetes, medications such as beta blockers used to treat hypertension, steroids used to treat autoimmune disorders, and conditions such as bulimia can cause elevated blood glucose levels.

Just as we can have fasting and postprandial (reactive) hyperglycemia, we can also have fasting and postprandial hypoglycemia. Immediate treatment of hypoglycemia and fasting hypoglycemia involves consuming high-sugar foods and drinks, and possibly medication, to bring blood glucose levels up. Postprandial hypoglycemia usually doesn't require medical treatment and is oftentimes solved by eating a balanced diet that includes high-fiber foods, whole grains, fruits, vegetables, and avoiding simple carbohydrates; eating several small meals throughout the day; and eating food while drinking beverage alcohol.

Given the information just presented, this begs the question, "Does sugar make kids hyperactive?" The short answer is, "No." If the pancreas is doing its job, blood glucose will be well-regulated. However, there is a persistent myth that candy causes sugar-induced hyperactivity. Double-blind placebo-controlled studies have found no correlation between sugar consumption and child behavior. Because individual variation does occur, these studies did point out that in *some children* (not the majority), sugar might have a *slight affect*. So why does the myth persist? It's likely that expectations affect perceptions. If you believe something to be true, then you expect it to be true, and thusly report it so. What likely is making children hyperactive after trick-or-treating or indulging in birthday cake is that this yearly event is something exciting and children are merely hyperactive about a change in routine.

We've spent a little time talking about the simple sugar glucose, but there are six sugars, scientifically referred to as *saccharides*, that are important to our bodies. Three of these six sugars are monosaccharides (*mono-* means one) and the other three are disaccharides (*di-* means *two*). Think of the monosaccharides as simple sugars and disaccharides as double sugars. Also realize that the suffix *-ose* means *sugar*, so any time you see a word ending with *ose* automatically think *sugar*. The monosaccharides are glucose, fructose, and galactose; the disaccharides are lactose, maltose, and sucrose. The simplest form of sugar is a monosaccharide, which cannot form any simpler sugar. Our bodies use carbohydrates first for fuel. Because monosaccharides are small molecules, they require no intestinal breaking down (digestion) and can be absorbed quickly, increasing blood glucose levels quickly as well. If you drink a sugary can of soda, glucose can enter the bloodstream at a rate of 30 calories per minute.

Yet, glucose is a simple sugar that is an important energy source. If you want to move, your muscles need energy and that energy comes from glucose. If your body doesn't need that glucose, then it can be stored as a bigger molecule called *glycogen*.

glucose + glucose + glucose + glucose + many more glucose → glycogen

Glycogen is stored in the liver and muscles and can be readily converted back into glucose if our body needs it. Glycogen is a water insoluble molecule and makes up about 10 percent of the liver's weight. From a practical perspective, the average liver contains about an 18- to 24-hour store of glycogen. The terms glucose and glycogen sound alike because they are both derived from the term *glukus* meaning *sweet* and both deal with sugar.

The reversible reaction in which glycogen can convert to glucose or glucose can form glycogen looks like this with a double-headed arrow to show the reaction can occur in two directions:

glycogen ⟷ glucose

Fructose is another natural, simple sugar found in fruits and honey. Without insulin, it is metabolized (converted) to glycogen. Recall that insulin helps move sugar from the bloodstream into the cells. You may have heard of high-fructose corn syrup (HFCS), a commonly used sweetener made from corn starch. To make pure corn syrup, like the kind you pour over your breakfast pancakes, the corn starch is broken down by enzymes into glucose. To make it high-fructose corn syrup, the corn syrup is further processed by enzymes (glucose isomerase) into glucose and fructose, forming a product that is 45 percent glucose and 55 percent fructose. Thus, many maple syrups on the market are generally just flavored with maple. However, some manufacturers are now using pure corn syrup instead of processed corn syrup because we're learning more and more about the long-term harmful effects of eating high-fructose corn syrup. A good lesson to remember is that the more processed a food is, the less nutritious it is for you.

What may surprise you is the link between high-fructose corn syrup and gout, the painful type of arthritis that affects the smaller bones of the feet, particularly the great toe. Inflammation occurs when uric acid crystals form in the joints. When the body breaks down fructose, purines are released, and the breakdown of purines produces uric acid. Gout was once known as a "rich man's disease" because wealthy people were the only ones able to afford foods—such as veal, scallops, red meat, and alcohol—which caused it. Today, it is a disease linked to high-fructose corn syrup, sugary soda drinks, and processed foods, regardless of sex or gender. Additionally, overweight people produce more uric acid than normal weight people, taxing the kidneys' abilities to remove it, thus it accumulates in the bloodstream causing gout. While there is medication to treat the condition, dietary management is a good place to start.

There is a degree of uncertainty within the scientific community right now as to whether HFCS is less healthy than other sweeteners. Whether the body handles HFCS differently than common sucrose (table sugar) is still uncertain. What is certain is that too much sugar of any kind is not healthy. Because high-fructose corn syrup is cheaper than cane sugar, it is found in so many foods that we consume and has been implicated in our obesity epidemic, increased diabetes rate, and increased prevalence of metabolic syndrome. Metabolic syndrome is a cluster of conditions—hypertension, hyperglycemia, excess body fat around the waist, elevated cholesterol and triglyceride levels—that occur together and increase the risk of heart disease, stroke, and type 2 diabetes.

Honey is a natural sweetener that has been touted for having health benefits. Research has shown that honey is rich in phenolic acids and flavonoids, two antioxidants that counter free radicals. (If you need a brush up on antioxidants, see Chapter 1.) Animal studies have shown that substituting honey for sucrose may reduce cholesterol, triglycerides, and blood pressure.

Honey is also effective for quelling a cough. Research has shown that honey mixed with warm tea or water is as effective as dextromethorphan, the cough suppressant ingredient in over-the-counter cough syrups. Coughing is the body's natural response for clearing mucus from your airways, so coughing can be good. However, if coughing is interfering with getting a good night's rest, suppressing it may be just what the doctor ordered.

Honey is not for everyone and should not be given to babies under age one because honey can contain *Clostridium botulinum* spores. These spores, commonly found in dust and dirt, contaminate the honey. If infants ingest the contaminated honey, the spores grow in their intestines, producing a toxin. This botulinum toxin causes botulism and infants have floppy movements, generalized weakness, and difficulty suckling and feeding. The condition can be reversed if recognized and caught early enough by intravenous treatment with botulism immune globulin, an antibody that works against the toxin.

Adults are not at risk from this type of botulism because the digestive system is mature enough to move the spores through the intestines before harm occurs. Adults and children are at risk for other types of botulism, including wound botulism from infection with *Clostridium botulinum* bacteria and foodborne botulism from eating foods—generally home-canned foods—containing the toxin.

Galactose is the third monosaccharide. It has the same number and kinds of atoms as glucose and fructose, but they are arranged differently. Galactose is less sweet than glucose, and it is a component of the disaccharide, lactose. Disaccharides form from two single sugar molecules. For example:

Monosaccharides Forming Disaccharides

glucose + galactose → lactose
glucose + glucose → maltose
glucose + fructose → sucrose

Lactose is known as "milk sugar" because it is found in mammalian milk, which is about 6.7 percent lactose. You might be wondering if lactose is found in human milk, why would so many people be lactose intolerant? That's a good question. People with lactose intolerance experience abdominal cramps, gas, and diarrhea after eating food that contains lactose. Common culprit foods include milk and ice cream. Lactose intolerance results from a deficiency of the intestinal enzyme called *lactase*. Note the suffix -*ase*, indicating that the term is an *enzyme*. Lactase is made by intestinal cells for the purpose of breaking apart lactose into glucose and galactose. These simple sugars can then be used to make ATP, the energy of our cells.

lactose (sugar) + lactase (enzyme) → glucose and galactose

Infants produce abundant lactase, which enables them to digest the sugar in breast milk and in some milk-based formulas. As we age, however, we may lose the ability to produce lactase. Approximately 75 percent of people worldwide do not produce lactase; but this figure varies by population. To illustrate, only about 12 percent of the U.S. population is lactose intolerant, but 80 percent of people of African, Asian, Hispanic, Indian, or Native American heritage are lactose intolerant. Tolerance—the ability to continually make the enzyme lactase and thus enjoy milk products—likely developed among early people who herded animals, drank their milk, and thrived.

Maltose is also known as malt sugar. In nature, maltose forms in germinating seeds; in the human body it forms when salivary amylase breaks down starch. Starch is a polysaccharide (*poly-* means *many*), meaning that is it made of up many sugars. Remember the simple experiment from Chapter 2 about placing a dry saltine cracker on your dry tongue? The cracker caused immediate salivation and you tasted something sweet. The job of amylase is to convert starch and glycogen into simple sugars.

starch and glycogen + amylase → simple sugars

When referring to carbohydrates, you also may have encountered two terms: refined and unrefined. Refined carbohydrates are found in highly processed foods, while unrefined carbohydrates exist in their natural forms. Diets high in refined carbohydrates are linked to increased risk of obesity and diabetes mellitus. Eating carbohydrates that are already processed means that the body doesn't have to do it, thus the body isn't expending much energy to break it down, so this step is already taken care of. Also, refined carbohydrates are absorbed much more quickly and lead to a spike in blood glucose levels, followed by a spike in insulin, then a rapid fall in glucose, and then you are hungry again. Unrefined carbohydrates release their sugar slowly so that "hungry again" doesn't happen right away.

Complex carbohydrates—commonly known as *starches*—are made up of long strings of simple carbohydrates. Examples of complex carbohydrates include starch, glycogen, and fiber. Plants store energy as starch, so wheat, corn, oats, rice, and potatoes are high in starch. Because they are larger than simple carbohydrates, they must be broken down into simple carbohydrates in order to be absorbed so glucose enters the bloodstream at a rate of about two calories per minute. They provide energy more slowly than simple carbohydrates, but faster than proteins and fats do. The take-home message: Complex carbohydrates increase blood sugar slower than do simple carbohydrates.

Dietary fiber, commonly known as "roughage" also comes from plants because it is a complex carbohydrate. There are two types of fiber, namely *soluble fiber* and *insoluble fiber*. Soluble fiber dissolves in water, while insoluble fiber does not dissolve in water. Soluble fiber feeds bacteria, so it's sometimes called a prebiotic. In terms of our diets, soluble fiber delays emptying in the stomach and makes us feel full. Insoluble fiber provides bulk as it moves through the large intestine and helps ease defecation. Insoluble fiber is sometimes called a probiotic.

Dietary fiber contains important chemicals like inulin, chitin, pectin, and dextrin, among others. You might see these chemicals on food labels, so when you do, know that they are good for you. Why are diets rich in fiber good for you? Fiber increases bulk, softens feces, and shortens the transit time through the intestinal tract. High fiber diets are also associated with decreased risk of cancer and obesity and lower incidence of heart disease and diabetes. Of course, high fiber diets and foods such as beans, are also associated with bloating and gas. However, if you eat a steady amount of fiber routinely, the excess bloating and gas usually goes away.

There are products on the market formulated to prevent gas. Two such over-the-counter products are beano and Gas-X, and each works differently. Beano contains the enzyme alpha-d-galactosidase which breaks down the fibers before they reach the colon, preventing gas. Gas-X contains simethicone, which is an anti-foaming agent that disperse trapped air bubbles.

If you also want to do a little experiment at home to test the fiber content of your diet, get acquainted with the feces in your toilet bowl after having a bowel movement. This isn't a grotesque exercise. Your feces tell you quite a bit about your diet. If you consume a high-fat diet, you'll discover that the poo in your toilet bowl floats; sinkers are indicative of high fiber diets. Corn is a special case: while one cup of sweet corn contains 3.5 grams of fiber, we don't digest all of the components of sweet corn. Corn—like celery—contains cellulose, and we don't have enzymes to break those chemical bonds. Hence, it comes out looking just like it went in.

In addition to vegetables, cellulose is also found in wood fiber, but we generally don't eat wood. The cellulose in vegetables forms bulk because cellulose is insoluble in water. In order for it to be digested, the enzyme *cellulase* must be present, and we humans do not have this enzyme. Hence, it forms bulk in the large intestine, aids in gut motility, and comes out pretty much in the same form in which it was ingested. Intestinal bacteria, however, do use the fiber. When intestinal bacteria break down fiber, gas results.

When it comes to nutrition, eating food is always better than taking supplements because real food contains vitamins, minerals, and other nutrients that are not found in supplements. However, if you have trouble eating enough fruits and vegetables, using fiber supplements is okay. At least there is no evidence that fiber supplements such as psyllium (Fiberall, Konsyl, Modane Bulk, Metamucil, and Serutan) or methylcellulose (Citrucel) are harmful. Like fiber found in food, they can cause gas and bloating, but their health effects still hold. If you're up for a fun experiment and you'd like to see how one of these fiber supplements adds bulk fiber in the body, take a heaping tablespoon of Citrucel or Metamucil and stir it into an eight-ounce glass of water. Then, let it sit on the counter for about a half hour and see what happens. You'll notice that it forms a sort of sludge. This is a good representation of what happens in the body when we talk about bulking agents and fiber.

Psyllium is a soluble fiber that absorbs water and becomes surrounded with mucus from the intestines, making it a good product for both constipation and diarrhea. It can also lower blood glucose and blood cholesterol levels, too. Methylcellulose is a bulk-forming fiber used to relieve constipation or to maintain bowel regularity because it is an insoluble fiber.

Diabetes and Metabolic Syndrome

We hear much about diabetes, but besides being a health risk, what is diabetes? There are three main types of diabetes and each has a different underlying cause. These types are *diabetes mellitus, gestational diabetes*, and *diabetes insipidus*. Our focus will be on diabetes mellitus and gestational diabetes because both are characterized by excessively high blood glucose levels that have a dietary component. We'll talk briefly about diabetes insipidus, but simply put, diabetes mellitus is a disease affecting carbohydrate metabolism and diabetes insipidus is a pituitary hormone disease. Yet, it's still a little more complicated because diabetes is a complex endocrine disorder.

Diabetes mellitus (*mellitum* means *honey*) involves insulin, the critical glucose-regulating hormone. With this type of diabetes, blood glucose levels get so high that the kidney blood vessels cannot reabsorb the glucose and it spills over into the urine, causing *glycosuria*. In fact, as early as the 1600s, doctors knew that tasting urine could provide clues about a person's health. The urine of a diabetic person tasted sweet, like honey. Although early physicians didn't know *why*, this early observation helped establish the foundational science for the disease. Improper regulation of blood glucose leads to excessive urination, which can lead to dehydration. The body senses dehydration, so thirst receptors are activated causing excessive thirst. These two conditions create the classic two P's of diabetes: polyuria (excessive urination) and polydipsia (excessive thirst). About 26 million Americans have some form of diabetes.

There are two main types of diabetes mellitus: type 1 diabetes and type 2 diabetes. In *type 1 diabetes*, sometimes called *juvenile diabetes*, the pancreas lacks the cells that make insulin. People who have type 1 diabetes must have insulin injections to live. In *type 2 diabetes*, sometimes called *adult-onset diabetes*, the body cells cannot respond to the insulin and/or the pancreas does not make enough insulin. Type 2 diabetes is associated with obesity, so generally the first treatment is exercise, weight loss, and healthy eating. With obesity, the combination of genes, inflammation, and other metabolic factors, results in tissue resistance to insulin. However, if diet and exercise don't work, insulin and/or other drugs to alter glucose synthesis and metabolism are necessary.

The third type of diabetes is *gestational diabetes*. Gestational diabetes occurs with pregnant women without a history of diabetes mellitus. It looks like type 2 diabetes, but typically resolves after childbirth. It still must be treated during pregnancy. Unfortunately, women who experience gestational diabetes are at increased risk of developing type 2 diabetes later in life.

Many clinical problems are caused by diabetes mellitus. The most common are diabetic retinopathy, cardiovascular disease, diabetic nephropathy, and diabetic neuropathy. Diabetic retinopathy is a disease of the retina causing vision impairment or blindness. Cardiovascular disease is widespread problems of the heart, blood vessels, and the tissues and organs supplied by the blood vessels, which is just about everything. Unfortunately, heart attacks are three to five times more likely in people with diabetes mellitus. Reduced blood flow to peripheral parts like the feet and toes leads to tissue death, ulcers, and infections—which can lead to amputation. Diabetes causes irreversible kidney damage, leading to diabetic nephropathy (*nephros* = kidney) and kidney failure. People with kidney failure can survive on dialysis, but this treatment is no walk in the park. Dialysis is a three to four times per week ordeal that lasts three to four hours each time. With dialysis, the body's blood is removed, filtered through a machine that takes the place of the non-functioning kidneys, and then the cleansed blood is returned to the body. Once a person starts dialysis, the average life expectancy is five years. Diabetic neuropathy refers to the nerve problems and nerve pain that results from abnormal blood flow.

In addition to urinalysis to check for glucose in the urine, another common blood test is hemoglobin A1C. Pharmaceutical advertisements for diabetic medication often mention hemoglobin A1C. This test is used to determine increased risk for developing diabetes, to diagnose diabetes, or to monitor diabetes. So how does this test work? This test evaluates the average amount of glucose in the blood over a two- to three-month period. It does this by measuring the percentage of glycated hemoglobin, which is hemoglobin with glucose attached to it. Hemoglobin is the oxygen-carrying molecule inside red blood cells. There are several types of hemoglobin, but one type is hemoglobin A, and glucose binds to hemoglobin A. This glucose bound hemoglobin molecule is now referred to as A1C. Once glucose binds to the hemoglobin, it stays there for the life of the red blood cell, which is about 120 days. Every day, new red blood cells are produced as old ones die and are cleared from the body. The new red blood cells are not glycated. But if circulating levels of glucose are too high, they become glycated. For these reasons, the hemoglobin A1C test is a good measure of glucose status over time. Here is a chart identifying normal and abnormal A1C values, which are reported in percentages. The higher the percentage, the higher the glucose levels have been.

A1C Percentages and Risk

A1C Percentage	Description
5.7% and below	Normal
6.4%–5.7%	Prediabetes; at risk for developing type 2 diabetes
6.5% and above	Type 2 diabetes

The last type of diabetes is diabetes insipidus. Diabetes insipidus is a disease involving the hormone *vasopressin*, also called *antidiuretic hormone* (ADH). Vasopressin causes the kidneys to retain water and increase blood pressure. With diabetes insipidus, vasopressin secretion is impaired or cellular response to vasopressin is impaired. It does share two hallmark signs and symptoms with diabetes mellitus, though: polyuria and polydipsia. So both produce large volumes of urine and the person is thirsty, setting up a vicious cycle of thirst and urination and urination and thirst.

You might notice that in science the term *syndrome* is used without any explanation. Common syndromes are Down syndrome, irritable bowel syndrome, and chronic fatigue syndrome. Syndromes are not diseases, which have a defining cause. They are not signs, which can be measured. So what exactly is a syndrome? Syndromes are a cluster of medical signs and symptoms or diseases which are not correlated with each other but are often associated with a particular disease. A syndrome associated with carbohydrate metabolism is metabolic syndrome. Metabolic syndrome is a clustering of three to five such medical signs and symptoms that includes central (abdominal) obesity, high blood pressure, high triglyceride blood level, high blood glucose level, and low high-density lipoproteins (HDL; the so-called good cholesterol). Metabolic syndrome is associated with the development of cardiovascular disease and type 2 diabetes. As a syndrome, its pathophysiology and exact mechanisms of development are still being studied. Research has shown that diet, body fat distribution, and stress play a role in its development.

Carbohydrate-Related Diets

Now that you've had a primer on how your body's cells use carbohydrates, let's delve into the various diets that center around carbs. Where to begin? There's the low-carbohydrate diet, the no-carbohydrate diet, the slow carbohydrate diet, and the ketogenic diet, among others. You may also know them as the low-carb, no-carb, slow carb, and keto diet respectively. As we discuss each of these, keep in mind the important role that carbohydrates play in cellular function. Also remember what happens when we have too many carbohydrates in our diet: we store them. These diets have one thing in common: they restrict the amount of carbohydrates you consume. Like every relationship, though, it's complicated. Which is another reason why diet fads continue to flourish. Restricting carbohydrates isn't such a bad thing, especially since research is indicating that carbohydrate intake has a greater influence on your general health than do calories. Think about that. The amount and type of carbohydrates play a bigger role than the number of calories in maintaining health. Not all carbs are created equally, and it is more important to know the type, quantity, and quality, keeping in mind that hardly any food only contains one type of nutrient.

A guide to determining whether a carbohydrate is "good" or "bad"—or better yet, which is "better"—is to look at its glycemic index. Numbered from 0 to 100, the *glycemic index* (GI) is a scale that ranks the number of carbohydrates in foods to show you how quickly a carbohydrate-containing food raises blood glucose. Glucose is given the value 100. Foods with high values raise glucose more than foods with low values. You won't find meat and fat on a glycemic index because they don't contain carbohydrates. Factors that affect the glycemic index in food are the amount of fiber, cooking method, and processing. Fiber decreases the GI while cooking and processing increases the GI. The basic glycemic index scale is given in the chart below.

Glycemic Index Scale

Glycemic Index	Value	Example Foods
Low GI Foods	55 or less	Fruits Non-starchy vegetables Oatmeal
Medium GI Foods	56–69	Whole wheat bread Brown rice Couscous

Glycemic Index	Value	Example Foods
High GI Foods	70 or more	White bread Short grain white rice Pretzels

One should use the glycemic index cautiously. It was developed in 1981 by Dr. David Jenkins at the University of Toronto as a tool to help people with type 1 diabetes determine the impact of various carbohydrates on their blood glucose levels. As such, you would think it a very valuable tool. However, there are some factors to consider. These same factors are those that make nutrition so complicated. Some factors include the physical structure of the carbohydrate, how it is processed, and what other nutrients (like fat and protein) are also found in the food. It's also possible to eat a low GI food with poor nutritional value. Potato chips fall into this category. Yet, a baked potato is a high GI food with good nutritional value.

Another consideration about the glycemic index is that we tend to eat mixed meals and don't eat any one food in isolation. Moreover, physiology is complex: protein-rich and fat-rich foods can release as much insulin into the bloodstream as carbohydrate-rich foods. The source of the protein, whether it is animal or plant-based protein, also influences insulin release. Evidence suggests that plant-based diets naturally regulate the optimum glucose levels in the blood, even when that diet is high in carbohydrates. The key here is the carbohydrate source and the level of processing, suggesting that whole food diets seem best at keeping obesity and diabetes at bay. David Jenkins even subscribes to such a diet that is rich in whole grains, fruits and vegetables, beans and lentils, with nuts and seeds.

What does a healthy diet look like? Healthy diets contain a good mix of macronutrients and micronutrients. Probably the most important macronutrient is water because our living cells require water for biochemical reactions. Per the American Dietetic Association, only about 45 percent of our calories should come from carbohydrates. With the low-carb diet, foods such as table sugar, bread, and pasta, which contain easily digestible carbohydrates are limited and replaced by proteins, fats, and very low carbohydrate foods such as vegetables. But are low-carb diets good for you? That depends. While we need carbohydrates, the American diet seems to have too many carbohydrates. Reports from the American Heart Association, the American College of Cardiology, and the Obesity Society concluded that there simply isn't enough evidence to make low-carbohydrate diets a staple across the lifespan. This is especially true for pre-teen and teenage years when growing bodies require nutrient-dense foods such as fruits, vegetables, and whole grains. Furthermore, in all individuals, if you restrict carbohydrates too much, ketosis can result.

Ketosis? Ketosis is a pathological condition characterized by increased levels of ketones in the body. Ketones are made in the liver when you don't have enough glucose. If you don't have enough carbohydrates from which glucose is derived, or if you don't have enough insulin to get glucose into cells, your body will break down stored fats instead. Basically, the body burns fat instead of carbohydrates. Your body can also make ketones after exercising. This is the premise underlying the ketogenic diet (keto diet), described shortly. With the keto diet, you burn fat instead of carbs and lose weight. However, if you eat a healthy diet, your body intrinsically burns the appropriate food source. If you restrict carbohydrates, the ketones can build up, leading to an abnormal, harmful condition called ketosis. Ketosis is marked by dehydration, confusion, and fruity-smelling breath. Ketosis is also a sign of uncontrolled diabetes.

Examples of other low-carb diets are the Atkins diet and the paleo diet. In essence, each restricts carbohydrates and stresses eating proteins and fats instead. Believe it or not, the ketogenic diet is the same as the Atkins diet—it's just rebranding, showing that diet evangelism is alive and well.

Ketogenic Diet

Let's take a deeper look at how the ketogenic diet works. This diet is rich in meat and animal fat. Remember that glycogen is the glucose reserve, but we only have about a few days of glucose reserve to draw on. So we need another way to obtain that precious sugar. One way is through ketogenesis. Breaking this word apart, we get *keto* meaning a *ketone group* plus *genesis* meaning *formation of*. Thus, ketogenesis is the metabolic production of ketones. If no glucose is available, the body will find a way to get a substitute source for our cells. That way is by metabolizing fats.

The organ responsible for fat metabolism is the liver. During ketogenesis, the liver breaks down fat into something it knows what to do with. This something is ketones. Yet we have these big brains that require glucose. Ketones are not the same as glucose molecules. So, if glucose supplies are low, the body can use ketones instead. This is an evolutionary adaptation to starvation when periods of famine outpaced periods of feasts. During famines, ketones replaced glucose and enabled our brains and other tissues to survive for a bit. But the body cannot survive long term utilizing ketones instead of glucose. In terms of long-term weight loss, the keto diet doesn't show any long-term results that were any different from any other diet. This is why "diet" should come to mean something that is healthy and sustainable for general wellbeing.

Another thing to consider is that while it is true that you will burn fat, low-carb diets also help you to feel less hungry. For the average person—that's likely you if you don't have diabetes, cancer, or aren't pregnant—ketosis can result in about three to four days of eating less than 50 grams of carbohydrates per day. In practical terms, that's the equivalent of one cup of low-fat yogurt with fruit, three slices of bread, or two bananas as your daily diet. Often reported side effects of the keto diet are fatigue, diarrhea, and constipation. These side effects can be short term. It's important to note that for the average person, a healthy diet with an appropriate level of exercise is always best, because you want to practice health behaviors that are sustainable.

Before you embark upon any extreme low-carb diet, be aware that ketosis can advance to a similar-sounding condition called ketoacidosis. Think of this as ketosis going too far. During prolonged periods of starvation or fasting, the body ramps up its fat breakdown for fuel use. Fat is the ultimate storage tissue of excess calories, so people can survive for days without food. However, as a weight loss tool, it can be dangerous because ketoacidosis can result. Ketoacidosis occurs when the ketones build up in your blood, causing it to become acidic. Acidic blood has a pH below 7.35. Normal blood pH range is 7.35–7.45. Anything outside this range spells trouble. In fact, a person has about 1 hour to rectify the low pH situation because acidic blood can cause coma or death.

In clinical practice, however, ketogenic diets might be therapeutic. The key here is the term *clinical*, indicating that a person is under the watchful eye of a health professional. Therapeutic ketogenic diets might help prevent seizures in children with epilepsy, and they may help people with type 2 diabetes and cancer. Although the exact mechanism for treating epilepsy with a ketogenic diet is uncertain, it has been purported that the keto diet makes neurons more resilient during seizures. Treating epileptic patients who don't respond to medication with the keto diet is not new: in the 1920s, researchers observed that epileptic people who fasted experienced fewer seizures. Stay tuned for more science to explain why in the near future. As for cancer, cancer is a beast unto itself and comes with a host of issues that are ancillary to the disease process, but starving cancer cells of glucose may enhance treatment responses.

Paleo and Ancestral Diets

Another popular carbohydrate-restricting diet is the paleo diet. This diet is based on eating foods presumed to have been eaten by early humans during the Paleolithic era, about 2.5 million to 10,000 years ago. This diet is made up of meat, fish, vegetables, fruits, nuts, and seeds. It excludes dairy, grains, salt, refined sugar, potatoes, legumes (beans, peanuts, and peas), and processed foods. The diet also emphasizes drinking water and being physically active. The thinking behind such a diet is that with the advent of farming, our genes didn't keep pace with our lifestyle, thus contributing to a mismatch between the food we eat and how we live. The premise behind the diet isn't so bad. Because it excludes grains and legumes, good sources of fiber and other nutrients have been eliminated, which isn't so terrific.

Not all the facts are considered with this paleo diet though, because diets varied depending on geography, climate, and resources. Archaeological research shows that wild grains likely were introduced 30,000 years ago while genetic research shows that the genome may have changed to accommodate starch breakdown. Let's take an evolutionary peek at our diet.

In order to understand nutrition from our physiological perspective, it is critical to view nutrition patterns from an anthropological position. That is, we need to understand the dietary patterns of our early ancestors, because the genes we have today are the result of a long history of feast and famine. We know that poor nutrition is linked with disease patterns. Interestingly, there is no evidence of nutritional deficiencies during the hunting and gathering era of human evolution, which ended around 8,000 BCE. Famine was unknown. Moreover, there was little food anxiety as 25 percent of the available food provided 90 percent of the diet. Our hunting and gathering ancestors had a great deal of respect for animals and there were a few ceremonies related to food. Yet, there was no fish in the diet until 20,000 years ago.

Diets of hunting and gathering humans were quite different from those of modern-day humans. Compared to today, former diets contained the following:

- 5x less sodium
- 3x more potassium
- 1⅔ more calcium
- 8.5x more vitamin C
- More vitamin E
- 2–5x more protein
- 10x more fiber. This fiber was mostly soluble, and the regimen was started in childhood
- No refined carbohydrates, and honey was used as a sweetener
- Fats were primarily polyunsaturated, but there were five times more of it in the diet

The issue of fat deserves some discussion. Ancestral diets consisted of a high fat content; however, the fat came from wild game. Wild game has about one-seventh the fat that domesticated farm animals have. Wild game is structural (polyunsaturated) fat, while cows and pigs have storage (saturated) fat. To illustrate, bison has one fifth the fat of a cow.

Acorns were also a substantial part of the diet. These acorns contained 28 percent more protein than the wheat consumed by modern humans. The nuts and wild beans of the time had high fat contents. Cereals, on the other hand, were only first introduced 15,000 years ago.

Plants found in the hunter/gatherer diet also differed. According to ethnobotanists (scientists who study the traditional knowledge and customs of people concerning plants and their medical and religious uses), the plants of yore had more fiber, calcium, vitamin E, and vitamin C. They also had a higher proportion of soluble fiber to insoluble fiber. This bit about fiber is important.

The general health profile of our ancestors was quite acceptable. If the person lived beyond youth, the life expectancy was good, and the average age was about 60 years. There was no obesity and very few were overweight. Other healthy characteristics included no high blood pressure (hypertension), low cholesterol and triglyceride levels, little tooth decay, and an efficient cardio-pulmonary system. Triglycerides are the main constituents of natural fats and oils; and high blood concentrations indicate an elevated risk of stroke. Today, we know that plant-based compounds like phenols, flavonoids, and antioxidants can prevent atherosclerosis, reduce cholesterol, decrease vascular plaque, and decrease vascular resistance (the force that must be overcome to push blood through the blood vessels).

Sweeteners and Added Sugar

A sugar by any other name would taste as sweet. Actually, it *might* taste as sweet or be sweeter as in the case of sugar substitutes. Humans like tasting sweet stuff and we have our primate heritage to blame. We evolved to eat sweet fruit for its higher energy and water content, and our tongues have taste receptors for sweetness. What isn't an evolutionary adaptation is thick waistlines that result from eating too much sugar and from not being physically active. That said, sugar, like much in life, is okay in moderation, consequently, it makes no sense to deprive ourselves of the little guilty pleasure.

Before indulging, a little perspective is helpful. Our cells do need sugar, but the sugar source matters as much as the quantity. We'll get into that. But before we do, here's a simple lesson on the various sugars. We consume lots of white table sugar, made from sugar canes and sugar beets. Other than calories, there is no nutritive value. When a food has no nutritional value other than calories, we refer to those calories as *empty calories*. Estimated calories needed per day vary by age, sex, and physical activity level, but for average adult females, the range is 1,600–2,000 calories and for average adult males it is 2,000–3,000 calories. Looking at white sugar, honey, molasses, and brown sugar, each of these varies in calories, but what still holds true for them all is negligible nutrition. Obviously, you'd have to eat a lot of sugar to come close to achieving any nutrition—and that would be at the expense of calories. Here's a quick chart showing calories and nutrient content for one tablespoon of each.

Food	Calories in 1 Tablespoon	Nutrition (Recommended Daily Values in mg)
Brown sugar	54	8 mg Calcium (Ca) (1,000) 0.2 mg Iron (Fe) (18) 3 mg Magnesium (Mg) (400) 31 mg Potassium (K) (3,500)
Honey	64	1 mg Calcium (Ca) (1,000) 0.1 mg Iron (Fe) (18) 11 mg Potassium (K) (3,500)

Food	Calories in 1 Tablespoon	Nutrition (Recommended Daily Values in mg)
Molasses	55	42 mg Calcium (Ca) (1,000) 1.0 mg Iron (Fe) (18) 50 mg Magnesium (Mg) (400) 300 mg Potassium (K) (3,500) 0.2 mg Niacin (20) 0.1 mg Vitamin B6 (2)
White sugar	46	None

Added sugars (sweeteners) include any sugar that is added to food or beverages during processing or in preparing. These added sugars can come from natural sources and include white sugar (sucrose), brown sugar (sucrose with added molasses), honey, corn syrup, and high-fructose corn syrup. Added sugar intake has been associated with increased cardiovascular disease risk and mortality among adults in the United States. Over consumption of sugar is also positively correlated with consuming more calories and gaining weight. The American Heart Association recommends no more than 150 calories (about nine teaspoons) per day for men and 100 calories (six teaspoons) per day for women. Most of the additional calories are consumed in sweetened beverages, namely soft drinks.

It's important to read food labels. It's really important to understand what you are reading because there are slight nuances in meaning. Here's a chart to help with the terminology.

Sugar Labels and Their Meanings

Product Label	What It Means
Sugar-Free	Less than 0.5 grams per serving
Reduced Sugar or Less Sugar	Sugar has been removed so that the product contains at least 25% less sugar than its original
No Added Sugars or Without Added Sugars	No other sugars or sugar-containing ingredient (fruit juice) has been added during processing
Low Sugar	Not allowed as a claim on food labels because it is not defined

The sugars on food labels are not broken down into natural sugar and added sugar. So, if a food has no milk or fruit listed in the ingredients and it has sugar, then the sugar it contains has been added. Healthy diets avoid added sugars.

Sugar Substitutes

Most sugar substitutes are non-nutritive sweeteners that make food taste sweet and contain no or low calories. Some sweeteners may be derived from plants (low-calorie) or synthesized chemically (no calorie artificial sweetener). Sugar alcohols, such as mannitol, xylitol and sorbitol, are derived from sugars such as glucose in cornstarch and generally not used in home food preparations, but they are found in many processed foods. You can identify them as sugar alcohols because their names end with "-ol," the last two letters of alcohol.

Mannitol is used as both a sugar alcohol and as a medication. It is about half as sweet as sucrose. Mannitol is good for diabetic patients because it is poorly absorbed in the intestines, so it has relatively little to no effect on blood glucose. As a medicine, it is an osmotic diuretic that pulls fluid from the eyes and brain, thereby decreasing pressure in glaucoma and intracranial (head) swelling.

Xylitol is a sugar alcohol found in some plant tissues and has the same sweetness as sucrose. Sorbitol is about 60 percent as sweet as sucrose and is found in some fruit like apples, pears, peaches, and prunes; and it can be made from potato starch. It is a nutritive sweetener and like other sugar alcohols can cause gastrointestinal distress in some people. Sorbitol can also be used as a laxative because it draws water out of the intestines, stimulating bowel movements.

Healthwise, sugar alcohols are good because they have little to no effect on blood glucose or insulin levels and they feed gut bacteria. However, many people experience digestive distress; but how severe the GI trouble is depends on the person and the type of sugar alcohol consumed. If you can tolerate sugar alcohol, it is a good low-calorie alternative to sugar. One thing to note: if you have a dog, be aware that xylitol is toxic to dogs, whose physiology mistakes it for real sugar. When this occurs, they begin secreting large amounts of insulin, causing glucose to move from the bloodstream into cells, causing fatal hypoglycemia.

Sugar substitutes are food additives and must be approved by the Food and Drug Administration (FDA) through GRAS documentation. GRAS is an acronym for *generally recognized as safe* and is a designation of the FDA that experts deemed this additive safe for humans. Chemicals with GRAS designation are exempt from the Federal Food, Drug, and Cosmetic Act (FFDCA) food additive tolerance requirements.

In addition to sorbitol, common sugar substitutes are aspartame, saccharin, stevia, and sucralose. The most common sugar substitute in 2017 was sucralose with 30 percent of the global market. Aspartame is one of the most scientifically studied and tested food ingredients with a high sweetness index. Sweetness index is a comparison of relative sweetness levels compared to sucrose; aspartame is 180–200 times sweeter than sucrose. Its discovery was accidental in 1965 by James M. Schlatter, a researcher for G.D. Searle Company. The story goes something like this: Schlatter was working on an anti-ulcer drug and accidentally spilled some aspartame on his hand. Later that day, while reading a book, a page was stuck. He then licked his finger and tasted something sweet. I have issues with the story for several reasons, namely, the researcher appeared not to be wearing gloves; he apparently didn't wash his hands after leaving the lab; and one never, ever puts anything in his mouth after working in the lab, particularly if he hasn't washed his hands. Nonetheless, aspartame was born.

Aspartame is made from aspartic acid and phenylalanine. Its trade names include NutraSweet, Equal, and Canderel. Although it was discovered in 1965, it wasn't approved by the FDA until 1981. Hundreds of studies have shown it is safe, is a suitable sugar replacement, and reduces caloric intake. There is one population who must avoid aspartame, though. People who are born with phenylketonuria (PKU), a rare inherited disease, cannot metabolize phenylalanine, which is a component of aspartame. For this reason, foods containing phenylalanine and aspartame must indicate so on the label in the United States. The label states "Phenylketonurics: Contains phenylalanine." Infants are tested at birth to determine if they have PKU.

Saccharin is about 300–400 times as sweet as sucrose with a metallic aftertaste. Its trade names include SugarTwin and Sweet'N Low. Studies done in the 1970s showed an association between saccharin consumption and bladder cancer in rats; however, further studies show no association between saccharin and bladder cancer. The mechanism by which cancer formed in rats was not relevant to humans.

Stevia is derived from the leaves of the *Stevia rebaudiana* plant. It is 30–150 times as sweet as sucrose (table sugar), but the purified extract is 200–300 times sweeter than sugar. Humans don't metabolize the glycoside building blocks of the molecule, so it has no calories. The plant has been used for hundreds of years in South America, Brazil, and Paraguay to sweeten tea and medicines. Sucralose is about 320–1,000 times as sweet as sucrose and is chemically made by replacing OH groups (hydroxy) on sucrose molecules with Cl (chlorine) atoms. Its trade

5

Those Are Love Handles

Lipids—Fats and Cholesterol

Dietary Fats

Fats generally get a bad rap. Some of the negativity is legitimate, but some it not. Fats taste great and they help make us feel full. Yet, like any diet fad that demonizes a particular food group, it is prudent to remember that we need all food groups. This means that you don't need to eliminate fats from your diet, you just have to choose fats wisely. Nevertheless, all fats are not created equal, but all fats do contain nine calories per gram—more than double the calories found in carbohydrates and proteins when comparing equal amounts.

Fats from food get broken down into fatty acids and glycerol, which the body needs for growth and energy. Phospholipids and cholesterol are used to make our cell membranes. Fats are also necessary to make hormones and to absorb fat-soluble vitamins A, D, E, and K. In order for you to absorb these vitamins, dietary fat is necessary. That means if you take a multivitamin in the morning, you should eat a little breakfast containing fat so that those fat-soluble vitamins can be used by your body. If we don't use the fats that we eat right away, they are stored as triglycerides in fat cells. And our bodies are really good at storing fat. Stored fat can be used when necessary, for those times when food isn't available, or if a person is unable to eat due to illness, or during intense exercise.

From a nutritional standpoint, they differ in their chemical composition and their effects on our health. You've likely seen various types of fats if you read food labels. As a rule of thumb, fats are labeled saturated, unsaturated, and trans. Let's think of fats in terms of how they differ chemically, how we cook with them, and what the differences mean to our bodies.

We store fat as adipose tissue, and this connective tissue has essential purposes in addition to making up our cell membranes, such as insulating us from the cold, and cushioning internal organs from bumps and thumps. It also acts like blubber on a whale, so it helps keep us afloat while swimming. Of course, that is dependent upon how much we have. The adipose tissue just below our skin helps with temperature regulation. However, the fat that surrounds internal organs is called visceral fat. *Visceral* is a word that means *organ* and having too much visceral fat is associated with cardiovascular disease.

Fats are the slowest source of energy, but the most energy-efficient form of food. To put this into perspective, let's take a look at Antarctic expeditions. Skiing across the bottom of the Earth, burning 7,000–9,000 calories per day in frigid temperatures hovering around -40°F, eating caloric-dense food is important. The food of choice? Butter. Slabs of butter are easy to carry, and each tablespoon contains 14.2 grams of fat. Carrying out the calculation, one stick of butter equals 113 grams of fat and 810 calories!

Like anything else, too much is not good: excess fat can clog blood vessels and accumulate in organs, leading to serious disorders. However, if you're skiing 12–14 hours per day across ice sheets, you probably don't have to worry about consuming too many calories.

Dietary fats vary in their chemical structure and it is this differing that changes what it looks like and how it behaves in the body. It's understandable that the average consumer is confused about fats because we oftentimes don't see the connections as there are so many names tossed around. A good place to start is by seeing the global picture, placing the various types of fats in a food scheme, beginning with common terms: saturated fat, unsaturated fat, monounsaturated fat, polyunsaturated fat, omega-3, omega-6, omega-9, trans fat, triglycerides, cholesterol, HDL, LDL, and VLDL, and matching terms with definitions. It is difficult to discuss each of these terms in isolation as they have overlapping chemistry. To put them all in perspective, look at this outline to get your bearings:

Fat

1. Saturated Fat
2. Unsaturated Fat
   a. monounsaturated fat

      b. polyunsaturated fat
          i. omega-3 fatty acids
            • alpha linolenic acid (ALA)
            • eicosapentaenoic acid (EPA)
            • docosahexaenoic (DHA)
          ii. omega-6 fatty acids
          iii. omega-9 fatty acids
   3. Trans fat
   4. Triglycerides
   5. Cholesterol
      a. HDL
      b. LDL
      c. VLDL

Chemically speaking, lipids, fats, and fatty acids are three terms for the same thing that are frequently used interchangeably. As a molecule, lipids/fats/fatty acids are made up of carbon (C) and hydrogen (H) atoms. Acids derived from fats are called fatty acids. Fatty acids occur naturally as waxes and oils and are found in animals and plants. Of importance regarding the various types of fats is the arrangement of the C and H atoms: these atoms create a hydrophobic (water-fearing) molecule that is soluble in organic solvents (mixture is evenly dispersed) and insoluble in water (mixture separates). In our everyday lives, consider vinegar & oil salad dressing versus mayonnaise. If we mix vinegar and oil, we can whisk the two ingredients together. It'll be fine on our salad, but if we leave the mixture alone for a little while it soon separates. If we want to keep an oil mixed in without separating as in our mayonnaise, we need an emulsifier. Emulsifiers help form stable mixtures because emulsifiers have both a hydrophobic end and a hydrophilic (water-loving) end. If we whisk water and fat, the hydrophilic end of the emulsifier molecule is attracted to the water and the hydrophobic end is attracted to the fat, creating a mixture that doesn't separate. In our bodies, bile emulsifies the fats we eat, creating little droplets of fats that enzymes can act on. Using an everyday example helps us understand that knowing a little chemistry is important to our everyday lives.

Fat in our food is generally a mixture of saturated, monounsaturated, and polyunsaturated. Foods from animal sources have a greater proportion of saturated fat to unsaturated fat and foods from plants have a greater proportion of unsaturated fat to saturated fat. Each type melts at a different temperature and the more unsaturated the fat is, the more liquid it is at room temperature. Now, we can take this a step further and look at the differences between saturated fats and unsaturated fats.

Saturated Fats A saturated fat is one in which each carbon (C) atom is linked by a single bond with a hydrogen (H) atom. They are called saturated fats because the carbon atoms are bonded to as many hydrogen atoms as possible, hence making it "saturated." Saturated fats, like lard, are solids at room temperature and come from animal products such as meat and dairy. Diets heavy in saturated fats are associated with coronary artery disease because saturated fats increase low-density lipoproteins (LDLs), or the "bad cholesterol."

Unsaturated Fats An unsaturated fat has one or more double bonds between the carbon atoms and where this occurs, two hydrogen atoms are missing. Two main types of unsaturated fat exist, monounsaturated and polyunsaturated, and the naming difference has to do with the number of those double bonds. Monounsaturated (mono = one) fats have one double bond and polyunsaturated (poly = many) fats have two or more double bonds. Unsaturated fats, like corn oil, are liquids and come from plant products. Figure 5.1 shows the molecular formula for saturated and unsaturated fats.

Monounsaturated Fats Monounsaturated fats are healthier fats found in oils and most nuts. Monounsaturated fats are "good fats" because they lower blood cholesterol levels and reduce the risk of cardiovascular disease. These fats also positively affect insulin levels and aid in controlling blood glucose in people with type 2 diabetes.

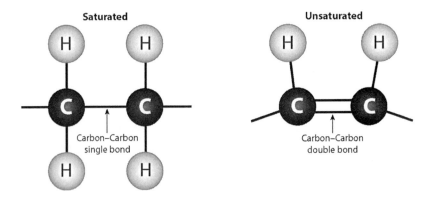

Figure 5.1 The molecular differences between saturated and unsaturated fats.

Polyunsaturated Fats From a dietary perspective, important polyunsaturated fats are the essential fatty acids. Essential fatty acids are called "essential" because the body cannot make them, so they must be obtained from the diet for optimum nutrition. Examples include omega-3 fatty acids, omega-6 fatty acids, and omega-9 fatty acids. These types of fats improve blood cholesterol levels, regulate blood glucose, reduce triglycerides, and help regulate blood pressure. Omega-3 fatty acids, found in fatty fish (especially fish with darker flesh), flaxseed, canola oil, soybean oil, and walnuts, play a role in lowering cholesterol and LDL levels, and they also have anti-inflammatory effects. Linolenic acid most commonly refers to ALA, alpha linolenic acid, one of the three omega-3 fatty acids. The three types of omega-3 fatty acids important in human physiology are the following.

1. alpha linolenic acid (ALA) found in plant oils
2. eicosapentaenoic acid (EPA) found in marine fish oils
3. docosahexaenoic acid (DHA) found in marine fish oils

Linolenic acid refers to a type of omega-6 fatty acid. Omega-6 fatty acids are precursors to endocannabinoids, lipoxins, and eicosanoids—all of which are being studied for their effects on human health. Omega-9 fatty acids are found in animal fat and vegetable oil. Oleic acid is an important omega-9 fatty acid found in olive oil. High olive oil intake reduces blood pressure because of oleic acid. Again, the names are confusing, but store these three in long-term memory:

omega-3 fatty acid = linoleic acid
omega-6 fatty acid = linolenic acid
omega-9 fatty acid = oleic acid

Trans Fats Trans fats, found in hydrogenated or partially hydrogenated processed foods, are chemically produced. Hydrogenation is a chemical process in which a hydrogen atom is forced onto a bond. It is done to chemically alter oils to make them solid at room temperature. Margarine was once created this way and we once thought this was healthy. However, we now know that trans fats increase LDL (bad) cholesterol and decrease HDL (good) cholesterol, which is discussed next. Trans fats have been banned in the United States, but some foods may still contain them in very small amounts. If a food contains more than half a gram of trans fat, it must be listed on the nutrition label. The USDA allows products with less than 0.5 grams trans fat per serving to list zero grams trans fat on the nutrition label. If you want to know if there are any trans fats in the food you are eating, look for "hydro-genated" or "partially hydrogenated" on the ingredient list. Eating too many (nobody really knows how much that is) trans fats increases the risk of coronary artery disease. We produce the necessary enzymes to metabolize saturated and unsaturated fats, but we do not have the enzyme to metabolize trans fats. Meat contains both saturated and unsaturated fats while trans fats are found in small amounts in products like shortening. For everyday purposes, we want to aim for eating more unsaturated fats versus saturated or trans fats.

Triglycerides Triglycerides, the main ingredients of natural fats and oils, are made from glycerol plus three fatty acids. Triglycerides are stored in fat cells just below the skin surface in our subcutaneous fat. When we have an increased level of triglycerides in our blood, the risk of cardiovascular disease is increased. Triglycerides cannot be absorbed in the small intestine (duodenum), so they need enzymes such as pancreatic lipase and lipoprotein lipase to break them apart into fatty acids and glycerol. Fatty acids can be broken down for energy or converted to other lipids. Once broken apart, the fatty acids and glycerol can now be absorbed.

Cholesterol Our bodies require cholesterol for cell membrane formation and steroid synthesis. In fact, cholesterol is the most abundant steroid in our tissues and is made from scratch by the liver from either carbohydrates or fats. So, regardless of your diet, if your liver is functioning, it will produce cholesterol—about 1000 mg per day. Cholesterol is transported as lipoproteins (discussed shortly) in the blood, reabsorbed, recycled, or if not used, excreted in feces. While cholesterol levels may rise with the amount eaten, it appears as though blood levels are dependent on individual cholesterol metabolism. Dietary sources of cholesterol come from animal-based food, but too much increases our risk for cardiovascular disease.

Cholesterol is necessary for the production of bile, an important salt that aids fat digestion. Recall from the beginning of the chapter that bile emulsifies fats. It is also essential for manufacturing vitamin D in our bodies and is necessary for producing the steroid hormones, estrogen and testosterone. However, cholesterol plays an important role in forming fatty deposits in our arteries. These deposits then occlude blood flow because they create obstructions to normal blood flow through the vessels.

Cholesterol is extracted from fat and released as lipoproteins, molecules made up of fat (*lipo*) and protein. These lipoproteins are reported as HDL, LDL, and VLDL, the abbreviations for high-density lipoprotein, low-density lipoprotein, and very low-density lipoprotein. Lipoproteins are very important because they are components of our cell membranes, and they form the fatty myelin sheath surrounding nerve fibers in the brain, spinal cord, and other parts of the nervous system. Myelin enables nerve impulses, and in diseases like multiple sclerosis, the myelin sheath has been affected causing disruption in nerve impulses.

The various lipoprotein names are derived from their densities, which are a ratio of the protein to fat. Here are the main differences among the various types of lipoproteins and why it matters.

Lipoprotein Types with Characteristics and Functions

Lipoprotein Types	Characteristics	Functions
High-Density Lipoprotein (HDL)	• Good cholesterol • High protein, low fat	• Pick up cholesterol from body tissues, transport it to the liver to be broken down and removed from bloodstream
Low-Density Lipoprotein (LDL)	Bad cholesterol • High fat, low protein	• Carry cholesterol to tissues • Carry lipids from the liver to other body tissues, but they contain a large amount of cholesterol
Very Low-Density Lipoprotein (VLDL)	Very bad cholesterol • High triglyceride	• Carry triglycerides and other fats from liver to muscles and adipose tissues

Blood levels of lipoproteins correlate with the risk of atherosclerosis (hardening of the arteries). However, it appears as though dietary factors are less important than heredity in maintaining appropriate levels of lipoprotein, cholesterol, and triglycerides. This is not true for all people, as some people do quite well by watching their intake of lipoproteins, but others can restrict fats and still have elevated levels. Moreover, other factors besides our genes can affect levels as well. These include diabetes mellitus, hypothyroidism, and liver disease—just to name a few.

High LDL levels lead to cholesterol buildup on the inner arterial walls causing blockages, hardening, and thickening of the arteries.

Arterial narrowing contributes to inflammation and leads to cardiovascular disease. *Atherosclerosis* is the medical term for this buildup and subsequent hardening and is derived from the word parts *athero* meaning *fatty artery* and *sclerosis* meaning *hardening*. Arterial walls have a layer of muscle and if the arteries become hard and thick, this results in stiffness. Stiff arteries squeeze inefficiently, preventing adequate blood flow, starving tissues of nutrients, and also possibly leading to blood clots. For these reasons, *high blood LDL* and *low blood HDL* are risk factors for cardiovascular disease. Other risk factors include hypertension (high blood pressure); obesity; physical inactivity; smoking; high-fat diets; and low vegetable, fruit, legume, and whole grain diets.

The Dietary Guidelines for Americans recommends that you get less than 10 percent of your total calories from saturated and trans fats, no more than 25 percent–30 percent from monounsaturated and polyunsaturated fats, and total fat consumption to no more than 25 percent–30 percent. For a typical 2,000 calories per day diet, 140–200 calories (16–22 grams) should be from saturated fats and unsaturated fats. To lower your LDL cholesterol, no more than 5 percent–6 percent of your daily calories should come from saturated fat. Grab a handful of walnuts and read on.

Diets Related to Fat and Cholesterol

Fat is a superior source of calories, adds richness to sauces and dressings, provides an excellent cooking medium, and helps the body make cholesterol. What is wrong with a high fat, high cholesterol diet? People with high cholesterol and elevated lipid blood levels experience a higher than average incidence of cardiovascular problems and certain cancers. When cholesterol circulates in the blood, it is attached to proteins of various densities in our blood plasma (the fluid part of blood), and plays an important role in the development of plaques on our arterial walls. Yet, cholesterol is a precursor to steroid hormones, which are important for normal body functions.

So what does diet have to do with cholesterol levels? It's a little complicated because dietary cholesterol contributes somewhat to blood cholesterol levels, but fat levels have a greater influence on cholesterol. Specifically, saturated fatty acids and trans fatty acids have greater influences on blood cholesterol levels than do cholesterol in food.

Restricting specific dietary nutrients is not a good idea. Thus, the so-called no-carbohydrate and no-fat diets are not prudent because our bodies rely on fats and carbohydrates. When fat is broken down for cellular use, carbohydrates assist the process. Without carbohydrates, ketones, the incomplete breakdown of fat, build up in the blood. While some ketones can be expelled in the urine, if too many build up in our tissues, the dangerous condition called ketoacidosis can result. Underscoring the point that all nutrients are necessary and human biochemistry is inter-related, remember that we discussed ketoacidosis in the previous chapter on carbohydrates. Ketoacidosis is that dangerous condition in which the pH of our blood gets too low. A key carbohydrate, glucose, has two routes it can follow: It can be used for energy or it can be converted into fat. When glucose is broken down into fragments, the fragments can be used for immediate energy. If immediate energy is not needed, the fragments can be reassembled into fatty acid chains which are stored.

Managing cholesterol levels in older populations is also a bit tricky: there is no one-size fits all recommendation. Research is suggesting that adding nuts to the diet is beneficial because their plant sterols can block cholesterol absorption. Nuts also contain fiber, vegetable protein, essential fatty acids, and other vitamins and minerals. It was once thought that nuts should be avoided if a person was trying to lose weight because they did pack a lot of calories. However, if nuts are eaten instead of foods such as potato chips and other non-nutrient dense food, they confer healthy benefits.

Fat calories are easier to store and harder to burn than carbohydrates and protein because the body preferentially uses carbohydrates and proteins for energy expenditures and stores ingested fat as fat in the body. Note, though, that the body requires some fat for efficient operation, tissue building, and vitamin utilization. This requirement is usually met by ingesting 25 percent–30 percent of the daily calories from fatty foods. Fats are caloric dense so if you consume a 2000-calorie diet, limit fat to no more than 600 calories (2000 × 0.30) or 67 grams of fat daily (600/9 calories per gram). In terms of food references, one teaspoon of margarine contains 11 grams of fat, one teaspoon of vegetable oil has five grams of fat, a small serving of lean beef or skinless chicken contains six grams of fat, and a cup of whole milk contains eight grams of fat. As is apparent, it is easy to consume a high fat diet, especially if the diet includes fried foods. Conversely, it is not too difficult to decrease fat consumption, but it does necessitate specific attention to the foods eaten. Keep in minds that one pound of fat contains 3,500 calories. Here are some guidelines for limiting fat in your diet.

- In addition to limiting fat consumption to 30 percent of the caloric intake, limit the amount of saturated or hard animal fat that is ingested. Be careful to read labels. Traditionally, convenience foods and fast foods are typically high in fat and cholesterol.
- Limit red meat consumption to three servings per week. Be sure to remove all visible fat before cooking.
- Remove the skin from the chicken before eating.
- Limit most fried foods.
- Used unsaturated oils and margarines for table spreads and cooking. Generally, the softer the fat, the more unsaturated it is.
- Use low fat, low cholesterol dressings and sauces.
- Limit hydrogenated fats. These fats have lost their "unsaturated character."
- Limit trans fats because they raise blood cholesterol level.
- Don't overdo fat restriction rules. Eat at least one teaspoon of fat in every meal.

What is the link between fats and disease? Fats contribute to obesity, diabetes, cancer, and cardiovascular disease. Cardiovascular disease is an umbrella term for a class of diseases that affect the heart and blood vessels. Examples of cardiovascular diseases are atherosclerosis and hypertension. We should understand that fats and fatty acids in food—not cholesterol—raise blood cholesterol levels. Eating omega-3 fatty acids reduces blood cholesterol the most, and these fatty acids may also delay cancer growth and development. It is estimated that approximately 90 percent of cardiovascular disease can be prevented through healthy eating, exercise, not smoking, and limiting alcohol consumption.

Butter or Margarine?

The quintessential question of our time is not "paper or plastic?" but rather "butter or margarine?" Butter is that tasty edible fatty substance made by churning cream (typically from cow's milk) until it gets hard and forms what we know as butter. Butter in your grocer's refrigerated section has coloring and oftentimes salt added during processing. Butter was likely made from sheep or goat's milk early on before cow's were domesticated. Early on, butter was made by hand as butter factories only appeared in the United States in the early 1860s. Butter was extremely popular in the United States until its popularity was displaced by cheaper margarine in the 1950s.

Margarine, formerly known as oleo or oleomargarine, is a butter substitute made from refined vegetable oils and water. Margarine was born in a lab when it was discovered by French chemist, Michel Eugene Chevreul in 1813. This is where it gets tricky. Typical plant oils are made of three fatty acid chains: two linoleic acids and one oleic acid. To improve margarine's texture and increase its melting point—making it good for spreading, keeping it a solid at room temperature, and allowing it to be used in cooking—these three fatty acids are modified through hydrogenation. Remember that during this process, hydrogen is added, changing unsaturated bonds to saturated bonds, thus the term "hydrogenated fat" is used for margarine. The high temperatures used during hydrogenation also change some of the bonds into a "trans" form, thus the term "trans fat." Tub margarines tend to have fewer trans fats than harder stick margarines. Since trans fats are linked to increased risks of cardiovascular disease, the food industry is working to remove trans fats; thus, some margarines have added plant sterols for their cholesterol-lowering effects.

Taking a step back in time, the advent of margarine was a scary event for dairy farmers who feared it would adversely affect family farms. The dairy lobby waged war on margarine and managed to get a series of laws passed, the first of which was the 1886 Margarine Act, that imposed tariffs on margarines producers. At one time, margarine was banned in Maine, Michigan, Minnesota, Ohio, Pennsylvania, and Wisconsin. Moreover, a law in New Hampshire mandated that margarine be colored pink. In 1898, the U.S. Supreme Court struck down that law citing that tinting the product pink "naturally excites a prejudice and strengthens a repugnance up to the point of a positive and absolute refusal to purchase the article at any price."

The question still remains: Do we eat butter or margarine? The best advice is to read the food label. Butter is pretty much butter across the spectrum in that it is made from animal milk and contains saturated fat. But not all margarines are the same. Some have trans fats, some don't. As a general rule of thumb, the more solid the margarine is, the more trans fats it has. Like saturated fat, trans fat increases blood cholesterol levels and lowers the good HDL cholesterol. It's a double whammy. Look at your overall diet. Your goal is to limit saturated and trans fats, so you decide on a daily basis where you want those fats to come from. You can also consider alternatives to both and use olive oil, avocado spreads, natural applesauce, or some other plant-based option depending on your purpose.

Chickens and Eggs

What about chickens and eggs? Are they okay to eat or not? What do cage-free and free-range mean? This is an area of nutrition science that has really been confusing for consumers. In order to be marketed as cage-free or free-range eggs, the U.S. Department of Agriculture (USDA) certifies cage-free chicken eggs and free-range chicken eggs by visiting the farms two times a year to check them out. So is there a difference between cage-free and free-range chickens and their eggs? Cage-free eggs must be produced by hens in a manner that allows the hens to have unlimited access to food and water and the freedom to roam during their egg-laying cycle. On the other hand, free-range chickens have all the luxuries of cage-free hens with the added bonus of having continuous access to the great outdoors during their laying cycle. Hens (female chickens) lay eggs regardless of whether there is a rooster (male chicken) in the area. For eggs to be fertilized, the hen and rooster must mate before the egg is laid. The mating ritual lasts only a few seconds when the rooster mounts the hen and their cloacas touch, transferring his sperm to her. This is known as the "cloacal kiss." The cloaca is the exit hole for feces and eggs and the entry hole for sperm; in roosters, the cloaca passes feces and transfers sperm. If a rooster does fertilize the eggs and they are incubated, they hatch into chicks in about 21 days.

Contrast cage-free and free-range with battery cages, the manner by which millions more eggs are produced in less humane settings. With battery cages, one egg-laying hen is confined to about 67 square inches her entire life. This is the minimum standard. Most eggs are produced by hens who live in such cages, unable to spread their wings. For perspective, a standard sheet of paper is 8.5 × 11 inches, roughly 93.5 square inches.

Digging a little deeper, we find that being cage-free and free-range isn't always pleasant, either. While hens must have access to the outdoors, it doesn't mean that they go there. The outside areas may be small and population density may limit their access or desire to go out. There is indeed a pecking order when it comes to birds and often they attack each other due to overpopulated living arrangements in what is essentially bird factories.

The vast majority of commercial chickens are raised under inhumane conditions. The lifespan of an average chicken is six years. Hens generally begin laying eggs around 16–20 weeks old. Like much in life, age takes its toll, and egg production goes down as they age. To get the most egg-laying power out of hens, farmers induce forced molting, a method of allowing a bird's reproductive tract to regress and rejuvenate. To induce it, food is withheld for seven to 14 days and water is also withheld for an extended time. Afterwards, the hen is ready to go again. This practice is common-place in the United States but is prohibited in Europe.

Chickens have natural molting cycles that are dependent on sea-sons. Chickens living in commercial farms cannot experience natural settings, so induced molting occurs. During the natural molting season, typically in autumn, hens stop laying eggs when their molting begins and start laying eggs again when their new feathers have re-grown. All kinds of animals molt; it's just called something else. For example, cats and dogs shed their fur, snakes and lizards shed their skins, and insects get rid of their exoskeletons.

Compare cage-free and free-range with organic eggs produced by hens that have access to the outdoors, cannot be raised in cages, and molt naturally. These hens also eat organic feed that doesn't come from genetically-modified crops and that doesn't contain animal byprod-ucts. Plus, antibiotics are only used in emergency situations for organic hens, whereas antibiotics are routinely used per conventional farm-ing standards with free-range and cage-free hens. If chickens are living in chicken factories in too-close quarters, they get prophylactic anti-biotics to stop the spread of infection. This practice is also discussed in Chapter 10 and is not good for human health because it leads to antibiotic-resistant strains of bacteria, which harms all animals, includ-ing humans. There are other options for raising animals in a sustainable way. They just cost more. If you are concerned about animal welfare, look for Animal Welfare Approved logos on products.

Have you ever wondered why there are so many different sizes and colors of eggs in the grocery store? It all boils down to the natural world as many factors determine the egg color, shell thickness, and size. For one, chicken breed affects eggshell color. You see this in the wild, too: robins lay blue eggs, sparrows lay whitish-gray eggs. The two most com-mon colors for chicken eggs are white and brown. The nutritional value is not affected by egg color. Nutritional value is affected by the hen's diet and environment. If hens are allowed to roam outdoors, their eggs con-tain three to four times more vitamin D than indoor hens.

The biggest factor in determining egg size is hen body weight. Bigger hens produce bigger eggs. All hens start with small, pee wee eggs and lay through stages that correspond with chronological age: medium, large, extra-large, and jumbo. As the hens age, the egg size increases, reaching full maturity around 40 weeks of age and maximum egg size at jumbo. Adequate protein level and feed intake lend themselves toward hens producing larger eggs. Overcrowding, stress, limited food, and inadequate water reduce egg size. It takes 24–36 hours to create one egg, and well-nourished, backyard hens who molt can lay up to 250 eggs per year.

Okay, I understand egg production now, but what about egg consumption? Currently, there is no recommendation for how many eggs you should eat each week. Egg whites are good sources of protein; but egg yolks have cholesterol and saturated fats, and we know saturated fat contributes more to LDL (bad) cholesterol than the dietary cholesterol does. If you are an egg eater, just be aware of your calorie count and nutritional intake. As a general rule for cooking eggs, it is better to poach, boil, or pan-fry eggs with cooking spray to avoid added fat.

Nuts, Dietary Approaches to Stop Hypertension (DASH) Diet and the Mediterranean Diet

Nuts were mentioned as a good food source for lowering cholesterol, and they seem to be the latest trend toward healthy eating. The reasons are numerous as nuts are a rich source of monounsaturated fat and are low in saturated fat; they are also high in fiber, vegetable protein, essential fatty acids, vitamin E, and plant sterols. Plant sterols are good because they block cholesterol absorption. While they do pack a nutritional punch, they are also caloric dense: half a cup has 130–200 calories with 80 percent provided by fats. Therefore, they shouldn't be added on to the diet, but used instead of crackers or other processed snacks.

We do know that diet, coupled with exercise, does have profound effects on both blood pressure and blood lipids, preventing disease processes, and generally lengthening life expectancy. Moreover, nuts are a component of two separate popular diets proven to control blood lipids and blood pressure. These are the DASH diet and Mediterranean diet. The Dietary Approaches to Stop Hypertension diet, known as the DASH diet, lowers blood pressure, reduces cardiovascular disease, and improves inflammatory biomarkers like C-reactive protein, which was discussed in Chapter 2. While inflammation is a normal beneficial physiological process in many instances, widespread chronic inflammation damages healthy cells, tissues, and organs. One measure of inflammation is C-reactive protein, a substance secreted by the liver and whose circulating level increases with inflammation. Therefore, if the DASH diet helps reduce inflammation, it has profound health benefits. The DASH diet emphasizes smaller portion sizes; vegetables (four to five servings per day); fruits (four to five servings per day); low-fat dairy (two to three servings per day); whole grains (six to eight servings per day); lean meats, poultry, and fish (six servings or fewer per week); nuts, seeds, and legumes (four to five servings per week); and sweets (five servings or fewer per week). Some versions limit sodium: up to 2,300 mg per day or up to 1,500 mg per day. This is a good diet.

The Mediterranean diet looks a lot like the DASH diet. People following the Mediterranean diet are less likely to suffer heart attacks, strokes, diabetes, breast cancer, and colorectal cancer. This diet is rich in nuts and olive oil, vegetables, fruits, beans, peas, lentils, whole grains, fish, and wine (especially red wine) in moderation. This is another good diet that is backed by solid scientific evidence and is discussed in greater detail in Chapters 6 and 9.

If you consider any trendy or well-publicized diet, be sure to include all nutrients in your daily food intake. Moreover, start using the term "diet" to mean *the food that you are willing to eat **regularly (not exclusively)** for the rest of your life.* Many people use "diet aids" to get them started, or to get them over the initial hump, or to lose those first 20 pounds. However, the reality is that we must engage in *life-long eating and exercise habits that promote health and well-being and graceful aging.* Thus, before you start any new diet craze, ask yourself this very important question: "Am I willing to eat such-and-such shakes and nifty-packaged meals that cost more than three houses in the suburbs every day of my life?" If so, get on the Internet and have your credit card handy. If not, continue reading.

As you can see, nutrition is complicated. The old thinking was calories in equaled calories out. While we know that dietary fat has more calories gram for gram than carbohydrates and proteins, each is metabolized differently. Don't misinterpret that sentence. This doesn't mean that there are certain foods that can get rid of body fat. That's not true. Some foods like chili peppers or coffee may boost our metabolic rates, but the amount is so small that it is negligible. Stay with me here. Some foods high in refined sugars trigger the release of insulin. If high-carbohydrate foods are eaten along with energy-dense fats, we're going to store that excess energy if we don't immediately use it. Like everything in life, moderation is the key. You'll fill up a lot faster on a bag of vegetables than you will a bag of potato chips!

Almonds and LDL

Speaking of potato chips, snacking is as American as pumpkin pie on Thanksgiving. A good snack is almonds for their possible LDL cholesterol lowering ability. Growing on a tree in a woody shell that we do not eat, almonds are the nutlike seed kernels found within. In a small study of 31 overweight or obese individuals who followed a typical American diet, researchers found some intriguing results: Adding one-third of a cup of almonds to the daily diet lowered LDL cholesterol by about 7 percent. The findings were reported in *Journal of the American Heart Association*. Although this was a small study, it shows promise for people struggling to decrease their LDL levels. In terms of dietary habits, it's easy to add almonds to your discretionary calories.

Almonds are a widely cultivated crop in warm climates, like California. What's interesting to note about almonds is that commercial nut producers have given funding to some government researchers to study the inexact method of determining calorie counts. The researchers discovered that cooking broke down cell walls in almonds, freeing calories for digestion. This meant that caloric values for almonds depended on whether the almonds were raw, roasted, or used for almond butter. These findings make sense because we know that cooking can also make nutrients more available, or it can destroy them. It's also interesting to review the methods of the almond study: participants were given meals with and without raw almonds and their urine and feces were analyzed to calculate digestible calories. What the researchers discovered was what many of us who examine our stool on a daily basis probably already know: sometimes undigested nuts appear in our feces. Thus, a serving of almonds has anywhere between 130 and 170 digestible calories. This discrepancy isn't really enough to matter when counting calories because almonds have so many other benefits. Where it does matter is in marketing for companies.

Cardiologists have focused on using drugs to lower LDL cholesterol. Popular medications used to lower LDL cholesterol include statins and other drugs, such as alirocumab (Praluent) and evolocumab (Repatha), for patients whose cholesterol was not controlled by statin drugs. What's interesting to note is that while drugs such as Praluent and Repatha lower LDL, it's not known whether they actually help people live longer. It stands to reason that mortality should decline because LDLs carry fat and create plaque on arterial linings, which disrupts blood flow. As of the writing of this book, more studies are needed in populations over the age of 80 to confirm the usefulness of lipid-lowering/cholesterol lowering drugs.

As for the statins, you've likely heard of the most popular ones because they are heavily advertised. They are also heavily prescribed. In fact, the most prescribed drug in the U.S. is atorvastatin (Lipitor). Other popular statins include simvastatin (Zocor), pravastatin (Pravachol), rosuvastatin (Crestor), and lovastatin (Mevacor). In total, these collective statin drugs have been dispensed to over 32 million people. That's a lot of prescriptions that were written. Yet—and this is a big one—recent research shows that these drugs had no effect on mortality and half had no cardiovascular benefits whatsoever. While most healthcare professionals will tell you how important it is to lower your cholesterol levels, that advice isn't being matched by the data.

There are no symptoms for high cholesterol, which is why it is important to get cholesterol levels checked. How often you should get your cholesterol checked depends on age. Via a simple blood test, HDL cholesterol, LDL cholesterol, and triglycerides are measured. According to the CDC, cholesterol testing should be done on the following timeline:

- Once between nine and 11 years (before puberty)
- Once between 17 and 21 years (after puberty)
- Every four to six years in adulthood

After age 40, your healthcare provider uses many risk factors such as smoking, diabetes, high blood pressure, sex, and family history in addition to cholesterol to assess overall health. Total cholesterol is the combined amount of LDL cholesterol and HDL cholesterol in the bloodstream. Cholesterol is measured in milligrams (mg) of cholesterol per deciliter (dL) of blood. Here is a quick reference chart.

Cholesterol Type and Values

Cholesterol Type	Normal Value
LDL (Bad) Cholesterol	Less than 100 mg/dL
VLDL Cholesterol	Less than 30 mg/dL
HDL (Good) Cholesterol	More than 40 mg/dL
Triglycerides	Less than 150 mg/dL
Total Cholesterol	Less than 200 mg/dL

Garlic and Blood Pressure

Garlic is a strong-smelling plant that is closely related to onions. It is frequently used in cooking to enhance flavors and as an herbal medicine to control blood pressure. A 2018 study found that garlic extract offers some benefit in lowering blood pressure, blood lipids, and blood sugar. Another study in 2019 showed some benefits for the cardiovascular and immune systems. In another study, researchers found that people who took 1.2 g of Kyolic aged garlic extract for three months lowered their blood pressure as much as blood pressure medication did. Normal blood pressure is about 120/80 and is measured in mmHg for millimeters of mercury; the top number is systolic (contracting) pressure and the bottom number is diastolic (relaxing) pressure. The garlic lowered systolic pressure 10 mmHg and the diastolic pressure 5 mmHg. This study also showed that Kyolic aged garlic extract also has the potential to improve arterial stiffness and inflammation.

Fish Oil Supplements

Fish oil is derived from the tissues of various fatty fish and contains the omega-3 fatty acids EPA and DHA. (Refer back to the chart if you need a refresher.) Taking fish oil supplements has been controversial for years as the research findings have flip-flopped. Current research is showing that fish oil supplements can benefit cardiovascular health, lessen the severity of autoimmune disease, and possibly ease dry eyes.

Randomized trials have shown that fish oil reduces cardiovascular events. The dosage was 1 gram/day for primary prevention in people who did not eat at least 1.5 fish or seafood meals per week. Another meta-analysis concluded that omega-3 supplementation at 376 mg/day to 4000 mg/day lowers the risk for myocardial infarction (heart attack), congestive heart disease death, and cardiovascular death.

Autoimmune diseases occur when the body mistakenly attacks itself because immune cells are not able to identify "self cells" from "non-self cells." Fish oil has been beneficial in treating two autoimmune diseases, lupus and rheumatoid arthritis. High dosages reduce inflammation, but there may be other mechanisms at play as well.

Slight improvement in dry eye symptoms were seen with nutritional supplementation with omega-3 and omega-6 fatty acids in fish oil. The evidence was not strong, so more studies are needed to confirm or refute findings.

Fish oil supplements can be found over the counter or by prescription. Prescription grade is guaranteed to be the real deal. Since supplements off the shelf are not regulated, consumers should look for the USP label or consult www.ConsumerLab.com, which provides ingredient analyses.

6

Packing a Punch
Proteins

Dietary Proteins

Proteins are quite important to our anatomy and physiology and their roles are quite varied, from forming structural components of fingernails, toenails, muscles, connective tissues, and skin to forming chemical messengers called hormones (epinephrine, melatonin, oxytocin, and growth hormone) to serving an important function as enzymes. In fact, most enzymes are proteins and their action in the body depends on their particular shape. In addition to these roles, proteins are active in immunity as antibodies to counteract specific antigens, such as those found in bacteria, viruses, or other foreign substances. Proteins also transport substances in the bloodstream. Hemoglobin is one such protein that transports oxygen, while lipoproteins transport fats. Proteins also have a role in maintaining fluid and electrolyte balance, and if too much fluid accumulates, *edema* results. The fluid of edema is mostly water, but protein and cells accumulate in the fluid causing swelling.

Dietary protein is an important nutrient that we need for growth, strength, energy, and so much more. Protein is made up of amino acids, simple organic compounds, that form long chains that are folded into various shapes. Some of these amino acids can be made by the body and some have to be gotten through the diet. How much protein we need varies, which makes recommendations confusing. Per the Dietary Reference Intake (DRI), a person on a 2,000-calorie per day diet should consume 0.8 grams of protein per kilogram of body weight. This is roughly 0.36 grams per pound, which equates to 56 grams for the average 155-pound sedentary male and 46 grams for the average 128-pound sedentary female. Generally, no percent daily value (%DV) is listed for protein.

Research shows that consuming 25 percent–30 percent of your total calories from protein boosts metabolism 80–100 calories per day when compared to lower protein consumption. Protein is also necessary to build muscle mass, which makes sense if you think about it because a good source of protein is meat, and meat is the muscle of an animal. Besides consuming protein, weight-bearing exercise also increases bulk muscle mass. With respect to gaining muscle mass, the optimum amount of protein needed cannot really be determined because individual diet, genetics, and exercise regimens are too complex. What is known is that people recovering from surgery or injury, older individuals, people with cancer, and endurance athletes need more protein than sedentary people. Again, there is considerable variation here, so the amount is dependent on the individual and can range from 0.45–0.65 grams per pound. Monitoring is key, especially in people with kidney disease, for whom protein intake must be limited. Protein can be found in both animal-based and plant-based sources; common food sources are beef, chicken, fish, milk products, eggs, beans, quinoa, legumes, nuts, and soy.

Necessary to all living organisms, proteins are one of the three macronutrients. The amino acids making up proteins are the building blocks of cells, and which amino acid gets made is determined by our RNA and DNA. Generally, our bodies use 20 different amino acids to make proteins that are needed for all physiological functioning and growth. These different amino acids occur naturally in plant and animal tissues and have the same structural "backbone" but have different side chains known as R groups. The amino acid backbone is made up of a single central carbon (C) atom, an amine group (NH_2) that contains nitrogen (N) and hydrogen (H), and a carboxyl group (COOH). Attached to the backbone is the R group side chain that makes each amino acid different from another. These amino acids can be arranged in a variety of combinations, so our bodies can make thousands of different kinds of proteins. Reversible reactions occur such that proteins can be broken down into amino acids and amino acids can be used to build proteins. Figure 6.1 shows some common amino acids and their structures.

The first amino acids were discovered in 1806 by French chemists Louis-Nicolas Vauquelin and Pierre Jean Robiquet. These chemists isolated asparagine, an amino acid found in asparagus. There are two types

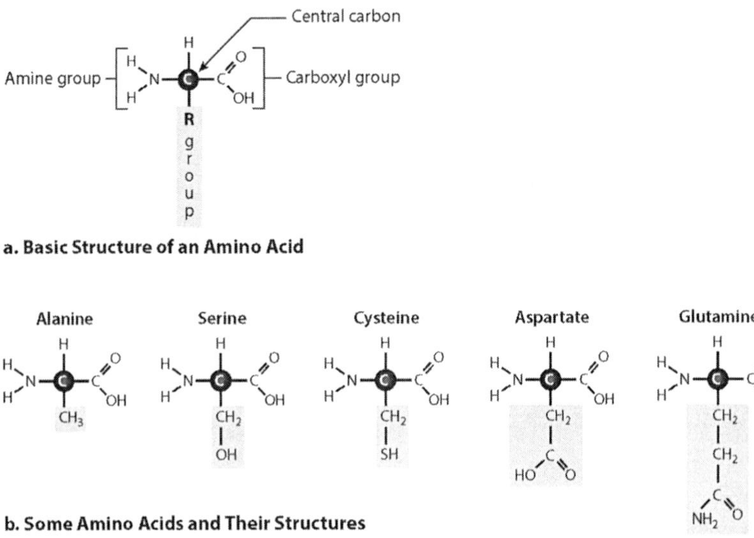

a. Basic Structure of an Amino Acid

b. Some Amino Acids and Their Structures

Figure 6.1 Important amino acids and their structures. All amino acids have the same backbone structure, but the R group side chain varies, creating the different amino acids.

of amino acids, essential and nonessential, and their naming seems a little backwards. Essential amino acids cannot be made by the body or they cannot be made in adequate amounts to meet physiological demand, so they must be obtained from food. Nonessential amino acids are those that the body can make from food. The human body needs 20 amino acids and of this 20, nine are essential and 11 are nonessential.

The reason that not all dietary proteins are the same is because different combinations of amino acids make up the protein in the food we eat. Foods that contain all the essential amino acids in adequate amounts are called *complete proteins*. Foods that are missing some essential amino acids or that don't contain enough in adequate amounts are called *incomplete proteins*. It is possible to eat two or more incomplete protein food sources, referred to as *complementary proteins*, to achieve the necessary amino acids. To be sure you get adequate amounts of amino acids, it's good to eat a variety of protein-rich food. Mix it up!

Amino acid biochemistry is complicated and beyond the scope of this book, but amino acids and proteins are central to our lives. The amino acid sequences along with their chemical properties determine what they do in our bodies as some catalyze (speed up) cellular reactions thereby controlling cellular processes. It's also difficult to determine the required amounts needed because so many factors, such as age, health, and activity, figure into the equation.

In order to read some nutrition labels or be well versed in the nomenclature, though, it's good to know the various amino acids along with their abbreviations. The chart below shows the essential amino acids and the nonessential amino acids with their 3-letter abbreviations.

Essential and Nonessential Amino Acids Important to the Body

Essential Amino Acids *Body cannot make them; obtained from diet*	Nonessential Amino Acids *Body can make them*
Histidine (His)	Alanine (Ala)
Isoleucine (Ile)	Arginine (Arg)
Leucine (Leu)	Asparagine (Asn)
Lysine (Lys)	Aspartate (Asp)
Methionine (Met)	Cysteine (Cys)
Phenylalanine (Phe)	Glutamine (Glu)
Tryptophan (Trp)	Glycine (Gly)
Valine (Val)	Proline (Pro)
	Serine (Ser)
	Tyrosine (Tyr)

To illustrate the centrality of amino acids in our everyday lives, consider monosodium glutamate (MSG), a traditional flavoring in Asian cooking. MSG is found naturally in foods such as seaweed, soy sauce, tomatoes, and Parmesan cheese. The compound is the sodium salt of glutamine (Glu), a nonessential amino acid. It also is responsible for the fifth taste known as *umami*, derived from Japanese and meaning *deliciousness*. We can taste sweet, sour, bitter, salty, and umami. It has been described as a chicken flavor or that of Parmesan cheese. We have tongue taste receptors that respond to glutamate, just like receptors respond to the other flavors.

MSG has been used as a food additive for decades, yet its use remains controversial. It is listed as a GRAS (generally recognized as safe) ingredient and the FDA requires manufacturers to list MSG on ingredient labels. Some people seem to be sensitive to MSG, triggering "Chinese Restaurant Syndrome," characterized by itching, hyperactivity, headache, and swelling after consuming food containing MSG. However, most studies fail to show any association between MSG consumption and physiological signs and symptoms. Even if the MSG intolerance is all in one's head, it is real for the person experiencing it.

Whether the proteins we eat come from vegetables, grains, or animals, they must be broken down into components the body can use. During digestion, proteins are broken down into smaller peptides, which are compounds made up of two or more amino acids. These peptides in turn get further broken down into single amino acid subunits. Amino acids can be used as energy, converted to glucose, or converted to fat. Unlike fat that is stored in adipose tissue, no energy storage form of protein exists.

Protein digestion begins in the stomach and continues along the digestive tract where a variety of enzymes act on the various proteins. Enzymes in the body denature the proteins, changing them into another form. Frying eggs is an example of protein denaturation: egg whites are liquid, but heat denatures the protein (albumin) in the egg white changing it into a solid. These specific enzymes break apart the proteins into peptides and individual amino acids, where they enter the bloodstream. In the liver, amino acids are synthesized into blood proteins, converted to other amino acids, or broken down further.

If heat denatures egg protein in a frying pan, does fever also denature proteins in the body? Yes, it does. Fever is a response to infection. Chemicals released by the infectious microbial agent, such as bacteria or viruses, induce the body's immune system to take action. One such action is to increase the body temperature above normal inducing a fever. The increased temperature can kill these microbes because they only tolerate narrow temperature ranges. (This is also the reason we cook some foods before we eat them.) However, if our body temperature reaches 104°F, cellular proteins are denatured, leading to cell death. For these reasons, fevers are advantageous, but can also be dangerous.

Each type of protein with its characteristic amino acid sequence determines what it does in the body. While this is determined by genes, our personal nutrition can greatly affect how genes are expressed. A classic example of gene expression influencing amino acid production involves the hereditary disease sickle cell anemia. In sickle cell anemia (also called sickle cell disease), the oxygen carrying hemoglobin molecule in blood is misshapen so that it is sickled shape instead of round. Blood vessels are long tubes that are just barely wide enough for traveling red blood cells. This sickling of red blood cells has two bad effects: It causes them to have low oxygen levels and it clogs up the blood vessels causing blood clots—the red blood cells stack up like dinner plates and stop traveling freely. Although we do not know if nutrition could ever play a role in influencing genetic expression in this disease, this example shows how one amino acid can make the difference between producing normal hemoglobin and producing abnormal hemoglobin. In sickle-cell hemoglobin, the amino acid glutamine (Glu) is replaced with valine (Val).

Here is the amino acid sequence (using the abbreviations from the chart) for *normal hemoglobin*:

Val-His-Leu-Thr-Pro-*Glu*-Glu

Here is the amino acid sequence (using the abbreviations from the chart) for sickle-cell hemoglobin:

Val-His-Leu-Thr-Pro-*Val*-Glu

Amino acids derived from dietary protein provide the substrates for protein turnover, the continuous break down and synthesis of body proteins using amino acids. Since proteins are large (complex) molecules, the body takes longer to break them down. Because of this, they are much slower and longer-lasting sources of energy. They are also the last nutrient source used for energy behind carbohydrates and fats. This means that if other nutrients are not available, as in starvation, proteins will be used for energy. During periods of starvation, the body goes into self-preservation mode, inducing important metabolic changes to maintain life. Most people reading this book have likely never endured prolonged periods of starvation; however, we all go through a shorter period of starvation known as the *starved-fed cycle*. This happens after we've eaten supper, didn't snack while watching TV, went to sleep, got up the next morning, and then ate breakfast. During the night, the body's goal was to maintain sugar balance, known as glucose homeostasis—a relatively constant range of blood sugar level to keep our body functioning. Our stored fuels keep us okay throughout the night when carbohydrate and lipid metabolism kept our glucose level where it needed to be. The starvation period was short-lived and we go about our day, only to pick up where we left off. And so it goes.

But what happens during prolonged starvation? For an average, not-overweight 154-pound, 5'10", 50-year-old male, initial fuel reserves total about 161,000 calories and the energy need is about 1,555 calories to maintain basal metabolic conditions. Basal metabolic conditions are real simple needs of the body like breathing, heart beating, digesting, metabolizing, and keeping warm. With enough drinking water, stored fuels can keep such a man alive for about one to three months, depending on activity levels. However, carbohydrate reserves are depleted within 1 day. In order to get the required glucose to carry out cellular functions, fats and proteins are broken down. Once the fat reserves are utilized, proteins become the main source of energy. Since muscles are made of proteins, this is one reason why starving individuals lose muscle mass and become weak.

The lack of dietary calories from the macronutrients and many/all of the micronutrients leads to protein-energy undernutrition (PEU), formerly known as protein-energy malnutrition. In addition to the overt wasting of muscle tissue, hair loss and skin atrophy (tissue wasting), also occurs. Because proteins make up our organs, multiple organs and organ systems become impaired, which ultimately leads to death.

At the beginning of this chapter, we learned that protein makes up our fingernails and toenails. Specifically, that protein is keratin. In addition to keratin, nails also contain the minerals magnesium, calcium, iron, zinc, sodium, sulfur, and copper. You may have heard that eating Jell-O or some other brand of gelatin will strengthen your nails. But is this true? It sounds plausible because gelatin, a flavorless, colorless, ingredient, is made from animal collagen derived from skin, bones, and connective tissue of cows, pigs, chicken, and fish. Collagen is a mixture of peptides and proteins, which get broken down into amino acids during digestion. The amino acids become part of the nutrient pool of the body, which do form structures like hair and nails and do play a role in building and repairing tissues and organs. However, nails are not specific targets for amino acids, but are part and parcel of our overall body.

Nail strength is affected most by environmental insults like hand washing dishes, working with your hands, trauma (accidentally hitting your finger with a hammer), and harsh chemicals. What is true is that infants have thin nails that tear easily, and as we age, fingernails get thinner, growth slows, and toenails get thicker. No nails grow after we die. If nail length looks longer post mortem, it is because the skin surrounding the nail bed has shriveled from dehydration, thus making the nails appear longer.

Meatless Monday and Concentrated Animal Feeding Operations (CAFO)

The importance of amino acids and protein is undeniable. Without a doubt, you understand that we need to eat protein, but there is a campaign to reduce the amount of animal protein in our diets. Enter Meatless Monday, a global movement encouraging people to not eat meat once a week. It was started in 2003 as an initiative of the Monday Campaigns, a non-profit organization working with the Center for a Livable Future and Johns Hopkins Bloomberg School of Public Health. Their goal is to decrease meat consumption by 15 percent with the aim of improving personal and planetary health. Check out their website at www.meatlessmonday.com.

Still, the history of "Meatless Monday" predates this 2003 campaign, going back to World War I and President Woodrow Wilson. Wilson urged families to help with the war effort by going totally meatless every Tuesday. He even took it a step further, encouraging one meatless meal each day for a total of nine meatless meals each week. The United States Food Administration (USFA) also encouraged food conservation as a measure to feed the U.S. troops and European populations where food was scarce on account of the war. The USFA was the agency responsible for feeding the U.S. Army and overseeing ally food reserves during World War I. The USFA's slogan was "Food Will Win the War." They also coined the terms "Meatless Tuesday" and "Wheatless Wednesday."

Meatless Monday also predates Oprah Winfrey's legal battle with the Texas cattle industry. In a 1996 episode of her show, Oprah was interviewing Howard Lyman, an animal rights activist, who focused on mad cow disease. At the time, mad cow disease was a growing concern in England. Mad cow disease, known formally as bovine spongiform encephalopathy (BSE), is a neurodegenerative disease of cattle and so-named because the brains of infected cattle look perforated and spongy. It is caused by an infectious, noncellular agent called a prion, which is a misfolded protein particle. Prions are different from bacteria, viruses, fungi, and parasites and are in a class all their own. In addition to mad cow disease, prions cause other neurodegenerative diseases such as chronic wasting disease (CWD) in elk and deer, scrapie in sheep (named because infected sheep continuously rub their heads against objects), and variant Creutzfeldt-Jakob Disease (vCJD) and kuru in humans. Cattle are suspected of contracting the disease by being fed meat-and-bone meal (MBM) that contained the prion. Note that herbivores were being fed animal-based products, a practice that continues to this day.

Back to Oprah. After conversing with Lyman, Oprah declared that this knowledge had "stopped her cold from eating another burger." And with those words, U.S. beef prices plummeted and ranchers blamed Oprah. Then, in December 1997, a group of cattle executives filed a lawsuit against Oprah, the jury trial began in February 1998, and by the end of the month, Oprah declared victory and maintained her free speech right.

Neurologist, Stanley Prusiner, won the 1997 Nobel Prize in Physiology or Medicine for his discovery of prions. All prion-based diseases manifest as mental deterioration, blindness, weakness, and wasting before ultimately leading to death. Should we be concerned about contracting a prion? We should be cautious. To date, the CDC has confirmed only twenty-six cases of BSE in North America. Six cases were in the United States and 20 cases were in Canada. As for variant Creutzfeldt-Jakob disease, it is acquired through eating contaminated meat. Kuru was first identified in Papua, New Guinea, in an isolated group of people who practiced cannibalism. The onset of symptoms may take a year or so after contracting the disease, so isolating the culprit isn't always easy. Unfortunately, there is no treatment or cure with death usually occurring within a year.

Fortunately, measures are in place to ensure the safety of our meat supply and protect against bovine spongiform encephalopathy. The Food Safety and Inspection Service (FSIS), a public health regulatory agency of the USDA, ensures that the commercial supplies of meat, poultry, and egg products are safe. For example, cattle that show signs of systemic illness and disease are not allowed to enter the human food supply. Under the FSIS's surveillance program, they are able to draw samples and test cattle for BSE. And probably of greatest significance is the fact that if something is labeled meat, it cannot include brain or spinal cord tissue. Keep in mind that this is for commercial sale of meat products. Animals that are slaughtered or hunted and butchered by private individuals are exempt. As a general rule, it is advised to avoid eating any animal meat taken from areas that are close to the spinal cord and brain.

Meatless Tuesday made a comeback under President Harry S. Truman in 1947 as he urged Americans to eat no meat on Tuesday and no poultry or eggs on Thursday as part of Poultryless Thursdays. The latter didn't go over so well, though, and the poultry lobby started "National Thanksgiving Turkey Presentation." Today, we know this as the annual "turkey pardon," when on Thanksgiving Day the current president of the United States ceremoniously saves one turkey at the White House. It's a presidential turkey pardon.

Meat consumption does play a role in climate change. Global livestock production creates more greenhouse gas than does transportation.

The phrase "less meat = less heat" pays tribute to this fact. Methane, the powerful greenhouse gas, is produced by cattle through stomach and intestinal (enteric) fermentation and fermenting manure in the field. Basically, cows burping, passing gas, and defecating contributes about 40 percent of the methane in the atmosphere. In addition to creating a disproportionate amount of greenhouse gas, livestock production uses 75 percent of all agricultural land on the planet and lots of water. To illustrate, here are some astonishing statistics related to producing one quarter pound beef burger:

- 425 gallons of water are used.
- The energy used would power your iPhone for six months.

Another area related to livestock production worthy of attention are animal feeding operations (AFO) and concentrated animal feeding operations (CAFO). Are you familiar with them? Here is a description taken directly from the United States Department of Agriculture Natural Resources Conservation Service's (NRCS) website:

> The U.S. Environmental Protection Agency (EPA) defines AFOs as agricultural enterprises where animals are kept and raised in confined situations. AFOs congregate animals, feed, manure and urine, dead animals, and production operations on a small land area. Feed is brought to the animals rather than the animals grazing or otherwise seeking feed in pastures, fields, or on rangeland. There are approximately 450,000 AFOs in the United States.
>
> A CAFO is another EPA term for a large concentrated AFO. A CAFO is an AFO with more than 1000 animal units (an animal unit is defined as an animal equivalent of 1000 pounds live weight and equates to 1000 head of beef cattle, 700 dairy cows, 2500 swine weighing more than 55 lbs, 125 thousand broiler chickens, or 82 thousand laying hens or pullets) confined on site for more than 45 days during the year. Any size AFO that discharges manure or wastewater into a natural or man-made ditch, stream or other waterway is defined as a CAFO, regardless of size. CAFOs are regulated by EPA under the Clean Water Act in both the 2003 and 2008 versions of the 'CAFO' rule.
>
> USDA's goal is for AFO/CAFO owners and operators to take voluntary actions to minimize potential air and water pollutants from storage facilities, confinement areas, and land application areas. NRCS can help landowners achieve this goal by providing technical and in many cases financial assistance, for the adoption of practices that will protect our natural resources.

CAFOs are meat factories that treat animals poorly, create breeding grounds for pathogens and subsequent diseases, and disregard the environment. CAFOs lead to infectious disease epidemics, antibiotic resistance, and waterway pollution. Something to think about when wondering where your food comes from.

Cooking and Cancer

Another consideration relates to cooking meat. It is true that eating a diet high in well-done meat and grilled meat increases the risk of cancer. But, do such foods contain cancer-causing agents known as carcinogens? When red meat, and to a lesser extent poultry and fish, are cooked at high temperatures, chemicals called heterocyclic amines (HCAs)—also known as heterocyclic aromatic amines (HAAs)—and polycyclic aromatic hydrocarbons (PAHs) form. The PAHs form when fat and juices from the grilled meat drip on the fire causing it to flame and smoke and then adhere to the meat surface. The concentration of these compounds varies depending on temperature, cooking duration, and type of meat. The mechanism by which these compounds cause cancer is not entirely clear, but there seems to be a link. We do have enzymes to metabolize HCA/HAA and PAH and perhaps the byproducts of this metabolism can cause DNA damage, contributing to cancer development. To limit your exposure to these chemicals, it is suggested to marinate meat first because this decreases the formation of HCA/HAA. Pre-cooking in the microwave also helps because it shortens the time on the grill. Trimming the fat off the meat also helps because this reduces flare-ups and smoking.

Eating processed meats such as hot dogs, bacon, lunch meats, and salami, has also been linked to cancer development. Some studies suggest that eating these meats cause the same cancers that have been linked to grilled and well-done meat. It's difficult to determine what's happening because it is likely that people who eat a lot of grilled meat may also eat a lot of processed meat. Furthermore, there is individual genetics to consider as genes may influence how the body responds to chemicals. Once again, this underscores the complexity of nutrition science.

Without realizing it, we really do use chemistry every day with particular importance placed on cooking, which itself is a scientific endeavor. Case in point is the browning of foods, known as the Maillard reaction. This process is a non-enzymatic chemical reaction between amino acids and sugars whereby once a particular temperature is reached, 280° to 330° F, foods begin to brown. With the heat comes many different flavors. The chemical reaction is a little sophisticated, but this process is not the same as caramelization, which occurs at higher temperatures and is a distinctly different process involving browning sugars. Examples of the Maillard reaction are golden brown baked goods, malted barley in beer, the flavor of roasted meats, and the browning of roasted vegetables. Experimenting at home, you can cook some carrots in a pan with butter. Until the temperature gets high enough for the Maillard reaction, the carrots will remain orange. Once the higher temperature is reached, the carrots will begin browning and the flavor will change. Food scientists have been experimenting with the Maillard reaction for years as they create unique flavors and artificial flavorings.

The reaction was first identified by French chemist, Louis-Camille Maillard, who was experimenting with protein synthesis. In 1912, he published a paper, "Action of amino acids on sugars. Formation of melanodins in a methodical way." Another chemist working at the USDA, John Hodge, figured out the mechanism of the Maillard reaction in 1953, writing about it in his paper titled "Dehydrated Foods, Chemistry of Browning Reactions in Model Systems."

A byproduct of the Maillard reaction is acrylamide formation. Acrylamide, a possible human carcinogen, was discovered in 2002 when scientists discovered that some foods cooked at high temperatures, especially food containing the amino acid asparagine, created it. Acrylamide is also used in industries including food processing and plastics, is found in cigarette smoke, and is found in higher levels in starchy foods like French fries and potato chips among other types of foods cooked at high temperatures. Scientists published papers on acrylamide formation in the Maillard reaction, and by 2014, systematic reviews of the literature were done on dietary acrylamide and human cancer. Many of these studies have been done on lab animals so acrylamide-to-cancer in humans has not been directly correlated. Several organizations, including the International Agency for Research on Cancer (IARC), the U.S. National Toxicology Program (NTP), and the U.S. Environmental Protection Agency (EPA) conclude that acrylamide is a likely carcinogen to humans. More studies are certainly necessary to determine if acrylamide in human food is linked to human cancer.

More Muscle, More Mass: Anabolic Steroids

Do you prefer white meat or dark meat? That is a personal preference. Is one type of meat healthier than the other? The short answer is probably not. The difference between the two types of meat has to do with anatomy and physiology. The color of meat is determined by myoglobin and iron content. Myoglobin is the oxygen-binding protein in muscles: the more myoglobin, the darker the muscle. Using chickens as an example, muscles that work harder, like leg and thigh muscles, need more oxygen. Thus, legs and thighs are dark meat whereas white meat is found in wing and breast tissue, which are required for short bursts of energy like wing flapping. Nutrition wise, both white and dark meat provide protein, niacin, vitamin B6, biotin, and vitamin B12. Dark meat contains slightly more iron and fat, so calorie wise, more fat means more calories. More fat generally means more flavor, too.

While chicken is the classic example to demonstrate the differences in white and dark meat, muscle fiber differences occur across all mammals, including us. Human muscles contain a mixture of muscle fiber types so the majority look pink. However, with athletic training, we can change the ratio of muscle fiber types—it all depends on what muscles we are working and how hard we are working them. The same holds true with other animals that you eat, which is why some animals like cows, that stand around all day, have a preponderance of dark, fatty meat. And now you know.

It is well established that meat is a good source of protein. When you eat meat, you are really just eating the muscle of an animal, many of whom have been injected with steroids to increase their muscle mass. Humans (think athletes) sometimes self-inject steroids to increase muscle mass and strength. So how does this work? The steroids used are called *anabolic steroids*, which are hormones that promote growth. The most common steroid hormone used is testosterone, a lipid-derived hormone made from fat. Both males and females make testosterone; the difference is that males make more than females. Muscle tissue has receptors for these steroids that cause muscle cells to produce more protein. With exercise and weight training, athletes bulk up as muscles increase in size. So the steroids bind to receptors causing an increase in protein production that leads to more cells that leads to an increase in muscle size. Here's an easy example: If you lift weights, each muscle cell in your muscles will increase in size and your muscles will enlarge. If you take anabolic steroids and lift weights, each muscle cell increases in size *plus* more muscle cells are made that also increase in size, so now you have more cells and more mass. It's sort of like earning interest on money in your savings account.

Steroids aren't all bad, though. In clinical medicine, they can help cancer patients and those on dialysis who are suffering from muscle wasting gain lean muscle tissue. But all steroid use—whether medically or illicitly—has consequences beyond muscle tissue growth. One such consequence is liver injury. Side effects of steroid abuse and misuse are lengthy. Some of these are high blood pressure, blood clots, heart attacks, stroke, decreased sperm count in males, excessive body hair in females, aggression, mania, severe acne, and jaundice. Animal studies also show decreased life span.

Okay, that's how humans use steroids. Now explain how and why steroids are used in beef cattle and sheep—the sources of human food. To begin, since the 1950s, the Food and Drug Administration (FDA) has approved steroid hormone implants to be used for growth in food-producing animals. Their purpose is to increase muscle growth rate. These steroids have been tested and shown safe for human consumption. The steroids can be purchased over the counter and are formulated as pellets that are implanted under the skin on the back side of the animal's ear. When the animal is slaughtered, the ears are discarded and not used as human food. Per the FDA, the steroid implant has a "zero-day withdrawal" meaning that the meat from the animal can be safely eaten at any time. Steroid hormone implants are not approved for use in dairy cows, veal calves, pigs, or poultry.

Steroid use in animals is controversial and studies are conflicting, which makes knowing what to do unclear. Just as in you and me, animals produce hormones, so steroids are present in all animal products, regardless of any hormone treatments. It's tough to know if steroid additives are totally digested or if we absorb some. Or, if the level of steroids we consume has any effect on our own endogenously-produced hormones. The FDA monitors our food and states hormones are safe. As a consumer, it's always best to error on the side of caution, so if you are concerned about hormones in your food, don't eat animals or animal products; alternatively you can buy certified organic meat and meat products and certified organic milk and dairy products.

Quinoa and Soy

While there are no such things as superfoods, if there were, quinoa might make the list. Quinoa, pronounced KEEN-wah, is an edible starchy seed that cooks up like a grain. It's prepared like rice and is loaded with nine essential amino acids. That's an impressive amount. Andean people have been eating the grain for 4,000 years and it remains a staple today. In addition to its protein, it is high in fiber and is a rich source of manganese and phosphorus. And quinoa is gluten free. Because of its superb nutritional count, ease of cooking, and potential for high-crop yields, NASA selected quinoa as an experimental crop for its long-duration space flights.

Much like quinoa, soy provides nine essential amino acids, thus it is an excellent protein source. Soy is also a good source of fiber, which helps lower cholesterol. It is also an excellent source of potassium with 886 mg/cup, which is double the amount found in a banana. Swapping soy for meat in cooking will lower your intake of saturated fat. The fat in soy is polyunsaturated and includes omega-6 fatty acids and omega-3 fatty acids, which research has shown are good for you because they lower LDL (bad) cholesterol by 4 percent–6 percent. Furthermore, soy has been shown to lower systolic blood pressure by two to five points.

Some research suggests that soy may help post-menopausal women build stronger bones. Soy contains plant chemicals called isoflavones, phytonutrients that mimic the female hormone, estrogen. Estrogen plays a role in bone strength, which is why some women take estrogen supplements after menopause when estrogen levels drop. The isoflavone may also protect against developing breast cancer in women and prostate cancer in men. Genistein and daidzein seem to be the isoflavones that protect against prostate cancer.

Soy does seem to be a healthy food for regular consumption. In some people, however, it appears that eating large quantities of soy products could affect thyroid function. The research findings are still confusing, so this is one area where we'll have to stay tuned.

Mediterranean Diet

Gaining popularity in the 1990s, the Mediterranean diet is a traditional diet of people living in Mediterranean countries, such as Spain, France, Monaco, Italy, Greece, and Turkey (to name a few of the twenty in southern Europe). The diet is characterized by eating large amounts of fruits and vegetables, legumes (peas, beans, and lentils), and olive oil; consuming moderate amounts of whole grains and red wine; and eating limited amounts of dairy, meat, and fish. Systematic reviews show that people following a Mediterranean diet had a lower likelihood of developing diabetes, heart attacks, strokes, and cancer.

Healthy diets typically include fish because fish tends to be a lean, low-calorie source of protein. Yet, we have to be careful how *much* and *what type* of fish and shellfish we consume because some types of fish have higher levels of mercury than others. Depending on where you live, you'll need to look at federal, state, and local government guidelines for safe fish consumption. The Food and Drug Administration cautions that large fish such as shark, swordfish, king mackerel, and tilefish are contaminated with mercury. If you choose to take fish oil supplements, tests have not revealed any mercury in the capsules. Yet, not all fish oil is created equally, it is not regulated, and some may be better than others. As always, if you are taking a supplement, be sure to look for the USP label, which ensures that the product contains what it is supposed to contain.

Mercury occurs naturally in the environment and is found in air, water, and soil. Environmental sources of mercury make their way into the water supply, contaminating water sources. Bacteria transform mercury into methylmercury. Mercury bioaccumulates throughout the food chain as fish and shellfish concentrate mercury in their bodies, and methylmercury accumulates as it builds up in adipose tissue. The food chain is a succession in which fish eat smaller organisms and bigger fish then eat those fish until predatory fish and birds eat those fish. Along the way, mercury accumulates, and some species can concentrate mercury up to 10 times higher than the species they just ate. This is called biomagnification because living organisms amplify the original amount. Since it is stored in fat tissue, it is not excreted. When humans eat these fish, we too absorb mercury, which also accumulates in us. Too much leads to mercury poisoning.

The health effects of methylmercury are dependent upon the dose, age or developmental stage of the person exposed, exposure duration, and route (inhalation, ingestion, or skin contact). Methylmercury is toxic to the nervous, digestive, immune, respiratory, and urinary systems. Exposure can also be fatal. In fact, the phrase "mad as a hatter" arose from mercury poisoning. Used by hat makers, mercurous nitrate was a chemical used to cure the felt (hair cut from the pelt). Chronic exposure to mercury vapors by workers caused mental confusion, emotional disturbances, and kidney damage. The medical term for the neuropsychiatric symptoms of mercury poisoning is *erethism*. Today, we know much more about mercury exposure, which is why we need to limit our consumption of fish and shellfish and why there is no mercury in childhood vaccinations. Taking tissue samples is the only way to really know how much mercury is in your body because blood, urine, and hair tests are not reliable sources for determining the levels. This makes sense since the mercury is stored in fat. People with high levels of mercury or mercury toxicity can be treated using chelating drugs that bind the metal in the bloodstream; after binding, the metal-chelator compound is excreted in the urine.

Eating canned tuna and salmon is a convenient way to consume protein and important fatty acids. But there is great variation among brands regarding how many fatty acids are contained therein. Moreover, many canned tunas and salmons contain mercury and/or arsenic (another heavy metal not conducive to human health), so they should not be eaten more than once or twice per week. Women who are pregnant, might become pregnant, or are breastfeeding and young children should be particularly cautious about consuming any such fish.

Atkins Diet

A popular fad diet with staying power is the Atkins diet. Started in the 1970s as a prescription for weight loss by American cardiologist Robert C. Atkins (1930–2003), the diet is high in protein and fat and low in carbohydrates. As briefly discussed in Chapter 4, due to its relationship with carbohydrates, it is similar to the paleo diet and other ketogenic diets. The diet has gone through several makeovers since its inception, but it still focuses on eating lots of proteins and fats and limiting processed carbohydrates. If you consume plant-based proteins and fats, the current iteration of the diet isn't so bad. However, if you have type 2 diabetes, heart disease, kidney disease, or high cholesterol, this diet gets a little tricky and requires careful monitoring with a healthcare professional.

A two-year trial comparing weight loss with a low-carbohydrate, Mediterranean, or low-fat diet showed that low-carbohydrate and Mediterranean diets may be effective alternatives to low-fat diets. People on the low-carb diet had better blood lipids and lost more weight while people on the Mediterranean diet had more favorably effects on glycemic control (managing blood sugar levels in people with diabetes mellitus).

Vegetarian and Vegan Diets

Yes, meat is an excellent source of protein. But if a person is not a meat eater (carnivore) and considers herself a vegetarian, will she be protein deficient? That depends. Vegetarian diets are as varied as vegetarians, but it is possible to get enough protein on a vegetarian diet. The merits of adopting vegetarianism include lower body weight, less disease, and longer life expectancy over carnivores. Various types of vegetarian diets include:

- lacto-vegetarian = person eats no meat and eggs, but does eat dairy products
- fruitarian vegetarian = person eats only raw foods and no animal products, grains, or vegetables
- lacto-ovo vegetarian = person eats no animal-based foods except eggs, dairy, and honey
- ovo-vegetarian = person eats no meat or dairy but does eat eggs
- pesco-vegetarian = person eats no meat except fish and seafood
- semi-vegetarian or flexitarian = person eats a diet centered around plant foods but occasionally eats meat

Of interest is that the 2004 term of the year, awarded by the American Dialect Society, was *flexitarian* because it was most useful in identifying cultural middle ground between meaty diets and vegetable-based diets.

Vegans eat no animal-based foods. Period. In additional to health reasons, many vegans choose this lifestyle for environmental (raising animals harms our planet and is an unsustainable practice), ethical, and compassionate reasons. Like many other vegetarians, they enjoy the same health benefits of living on this planet longer with fewer diseases. A note of caution, however: Animals or animal products are the only source of vitamin B12, so strict vegan diets will lead to a vitamin B12 deficiency without supplements (pills, injections, or fortified foods) of some sort.

Some of the latest research shows that plant-based diets have health advantages compared to animal-protein based diets. These health advantages include living longer, less heart disease, lower risk of cancer, and a lower likelihood of getting type 2 diabetes. Diets rich in vegetables (without fattening sauces), fruits, whole grains, legumes, and nuts seem to be protective against disease. Foods we should try to avoid—or at the very least limit—include refined grains, processed foods, and sweetened drinks.

As I write, Burger King has placed the Impossible Burger on its menu. The Impossible Burger is a plant-based food that tastes like ground beef and has been made in the lab. Other plant-based foods have been synthesized in the lab, too, including an array from Beyond Meat. Having just described how plant-based diets are beneficial to health, it stands to reason that this sandwich food would be good for you. But is it? While the way in which it is manufactured may be better for the planet and satisfy the no-kill rule for animal lovers, this is still a highly processed food. And as a newcomer on the market, there are not enough scientific studies to confirm or dispute its overall healthiness for consumption. That said, the manufacturer's goal was not to make healthier burgers. Their goal was to make something that had a less deleterious impact on the environment while providing people with the taste of real meat.

Traditional meat companies, including Tyson, Smithfield, Perdue, Hormel, and Nestle, have also gotten on the meatless, plant-based, or meat-plant mixture wagon. We can now buy plant-based burgers, meatballs, and chicken nuggets from these meat conglomerates. Again, time will tell whether these are truly healthy alternatives or not.

Blood Type Diet

There are four main blood types found among humans: Type A, Type B, Type AB, and Type O. Your blood type is genetically determined and inherited from a combination of genes from both parents. The letters indicate the presence (A, B, AB) or absence (O) of surface proteins called antigens on the red blood cells. See Figure 6.2 to view the various red blood cells with their surface antigens.

The blood type diet is another fad diet based on the notion that distinct diets benefit particular blood types and has to do with lectins. Lectins are carbohydrate-binding proteins. To date there is no scientific evidence supporting its underlying premise that people with different blood types digest lectins differently. The link between lectins and blood type lies in the test for blood types itself: Glycolipids and glycoproteins, found on the surface of red blood cells, can be identified by lectins. In terms of diet, lectins are found in many protein-containing foods and

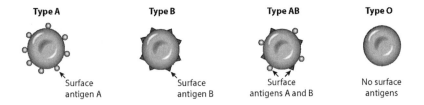

Figure 6.2 Blood types. The presence or absence of a surface antigen on the red blood cell determines a person's blood type.

using your imagination, different diets are recommended given your blood type and its lectins. Stick with me here.

In 1996, naturopathic physician Peter D'Adamo wrote the book *Eat Right for Your Type*. It provides recommendations for particular diets depending on your blood type. It has been revised and updated and is achieving great success. The underlying science is non-existent, and the diet myths have been debunked numerous times. Here's a rundown of the basics per the four blood types.

> *Blood Type A*
> Eat: fruit, vegetables, tofu, seafood, turkey, and whole grains
> Avoid: meat
>
> *Blood Type B*
> Eat: a diverse diet with meat, fruit, dairy, seafood, and grains
> Avoid: chicken, corn, peanuts, and wheat
>
> *Blood Type AB*
> Eat: dairy, tofu, lamb, fish, grains, fruits, and vegetables
> Avoid: chicken, corn, buckwheat, and kidney beans
>
> *Blood Type O*
> Eat: high protein food, lots of meat, fruit, vegetables, and fish
> Limit: grains, beans, legumes

In 2018, the British Dietetic Association (BDA) named the blood type diet as the number one "Top 5 Celeb Diets to Avoid in 2019." In case you were curious, here are the diets rounding out that list.

> #2: Drinking Your Own Pee
> #3: Detox Teas/Skinny Coffee
> #4: Slimming Sachets
> #5: Alkaline Water

The BDA sums up these diets as "endless fads, endless sales opportunities." Science couldn't agree more.

That brings us to lectin-free diets. Lectin-free diets exclude grains, legumes, eggs, and many fruits and vegetables—the very foods that research has shown to be beneficial. The diet gained popularity by Steven Gundry, an American cardiac surgeon and author of *The Plant Paradox: The Hidden Dangers in "Healthy" Foods That Cause Disease and Weight Gain*. And this is where science gets messy. Not only is Dr. Gundry a best-selling author and pioneer in heart transplant surgery, he peddles supplements and pseudoscience.

Amino Acid Supplements

Nature provides all the protein we need to eat to stay healthy. Yet, many people will want to consume high-protein diets, protein supplements, and/or amino acid supplements. As we've established, how much protein a person needs depends on the person's health status, body size, activity level, and stage in life.

The value of amino acid supplementation in clinical medicine is still under investigation, particularly in treating cachexia and sarcopenia. Cachexia is a complex syndrome characterized by weakness and muscle wasting that results from severe chronic illness such as cancer and AIDS. Sarcopenia is the loss of skeletal muscle mass whose rate is dependent upon exercise level, co-morbidities, and nutrition. It's difficult to see the differences between cachexia and sarcopenia because outwardly they look the same; however, the underlying biochemical pathways leading to each is different. Nonetheless, both conditions can co-exist. It stands to reason that supplementing with amino acids and protein should be beneficial for cachexia, but treating cachexia with supplementation has shown little to no benefit without eradicating the underlying illness.

For the average person, the value of protein supplements and amino acid supplements have not been borne out in the scientific literature. There are few published papers that deal with the safe upper limits or toxicity level for amino acid supplements in healthy people. While we know the role of amino acids for many biological processes and pathological conditions, genetic expression and other factors may play a role in determining the effectiveness of amino acid supplementation.

7

Alphabet Soup
and Dietary Mining
Vitamins and Minerals

Micronutrients

Micronutrients are vitamins and minerals. This means that you need them in very small (micro) amounts for normal physiological function, growth and development, and good nutrition. By their nature, vitamins are organic substances, meaning they contain carbon, while minerals are inorganic elements, meaning they do not contain carbon. The word *vitamin* is derived from the Latin term *vita* that means *life* + *amine* that means *amino acid*. This is a bit confusing because there are no amino acids in vitamins; they were originally thought to contain amino acids. Vegetables contain various vitamins and minerals, so they should be part of our daily diets. You might be thinking, which is better—raw or cooked? Whether or not raw vegetables are better for you depends on the vegetable and the method of cooking. For example, some vitamins in foods are lost through cooking and others become more bioavailable (usable) to the body when they are cooked. Remembering which vegetables are better raw or cooked isn't necessary because the key is to make sure you get heaping helpings of their goodness daily.

When we look at the makeup of the human body, we are made of many elements and compounds, most of which is water, H_2O. In fact, the majority of the body's mass is hydrogen (H) and oxygen (O), which combine to form that water and thereby create a lot of mass. As single elements, hydrogen and oxygen don't weigh that much, but put them together to form water and that changes dramatically as anybody moving a child's wading pool can tell you. Water in the body gives us most of our mass, too. Of all the elements in the universe, approximately 99 percent of the body's mass is made up of just six major elements: oxygen, carbon, hydrogen, nitrogen, calcium, and phosphorus. However, oxygen, carbon, hydrogen, and nitrogen are not listed as major nutrients that you must obtain from the diet. You might *get them* from your diet as you consume food that contains them, but they are not necessary for vital body functions. A plant may take up some nutrient from the soil and when we eat that plant, the nutrient becomes part of us, hanging out in body tissues. For an idea of the various elements within the body, take a look at the chart below that gives the breakdown of the body's composition.

Elements of the Human Body

Element	Approximate Percentage (%)
Oxygen (O)	65%
Carbon (C)	18%
Hydrogen (H)	10%
Nitrogen (N)	3%
Calcium (Ca)	1.5%
Phosphorus (P)	1.0%
Potassium (K)	0.35%
Sulfur (S)	0.25%
Sodium (Na)	0.15%
Chlorine (Cl)	0.15%
Magnesium (Mg)	0.05%
Iron (Fe)	0.006%
Copper (Cu), Zinc (Z), Selenium (Se), Molybdenum (Mo), Fluorine (F), Iodine (I), Manganese (Mn), Cobalt (Co)	Total less than 0.50%
Lithium (Li), Strontium (Sr), Aluminum (Al), Silicon (Si), Lead (Pb), Vanadium (V), Arsenic (As), Bromine (B)	Present in trace amounts
Molecules (95%)	Approximate Percentage (%)
Water	62%
Protein	16%
Fat	16%
Carbohydrate	1%

Water-Soluble Vitamins

Let's begin with vitamins, those little organic substances that are not synthesized in the body and must be obtained from the food we eat in some fashion. This means that either the food has the actual vitamin we need, or the food feeds some gut bacteria that make the vitamin. Examples of vitamins made by gut bacteria include most of the B vitamins and vitamin K. An important function of vitamins is to serve as coenzymes aiding the function of another enzyme. Remember from our previous discussion on protein that most enzymes are proteins; vitamins can assist protein function.

There are two types of vitamins, based on their ability to dissolve: water-soluble and fat-soluble. We talked about fat-soluble vitamins in Chapter 5 when we discussed the importance of fat in the diet because fat enables the absorption of the fat-soluble vitamins, namely A, D, E, and K. Water-soluble vitamins dissolve in water and don't need fat to be absorbed. Examples of water-soluble vitamins are the variety of B complex vitamins and vitamin C. These vitamins all have alternate names, and you're probably familiar with lots of them. Here's the laundry list:

- thiamin (vitamin B1)
- riboflavin (vitamin B2)
- niacin (vitamin B3)
- pantothenic acid (vitamin B5)
- pyridoxine (vitamin B6)
- biotin (vitamin B7)
- folic acid (vitamin B9)
- cobalamin (vitamin B12)
- ascorbic acid (vitamin C)

A chart showing the water-soluble vitamins and their common names, listing their importance, food sources, and the effects of excess and deficiency is given below. Water-soluble vitamins are easily exchanged between the fluid compartments of the digestive tract and the bloodstream. Since the body is an interplay of several body systems, fluid balance is achieved through the functions of many systems working together. One such system is the urinary system, where the kidneys play a major role in achieving water-soluble vitamin balance. The kidneys have an upper limit (threshold) of how much water-soluble vitamins they can process so any excesses are excreted in the urine. For this reason, if you take water-soluble vitamin supplements in an amount greater than the kidney threshold, they will wind up in your toilet bowl instead of your body. This is also why it is difficult to over-indulge in water-soluble vitamins: Excesses will be excreted in urine. Although rare, it *can* happen, especially if larger quantities of vitamins are taken in a short period of time.

An excessive consumption of vitamins, or vitamin overdose, causes a condition known as hypervitaminosis. *Hyper-* means too much, and *-osis* means condition. How much is too much? The United States Department of Agriculture (USDA) defines "tolerable upper intake level" for vitamins and lists them under its Dietary Reference Intake (DRI). Vitamin overdose rarely occurs from eating food, but it can occur with vitamin supplementation. Two fat-soluble vitamins that can lead to hypervitaminosis are vitamin A and vitamin D. A recent Annual Report of the American Association of Poison Control Centers' National Poison Data System (NPDS) reported 59,761 individuals with overdose exposure to all formulations of vitamins and multi-vitamin/mineral supplements with 42,553 of these exposures in children aged 5 and under. In nearly all instances—excepting disease states and special conditions of the person—vitamin and mineral supplementation is unnecessary as balanced diets can provide all the nutrients and quantities we need.

Water-Soluble Vitamins Chart

Vitamin Alternate Name • Food Sources	Importance	Effects of Excessiveness	Effects of Deficiency
B1 Thiamine • Milk, yeast, grains	Coenzyme in metabolic pathways	Low blood pressure (hypotension)	Muscle weakness, cardiovascular problems
B2 Riboflavin • Green vegetables, liver, kidneys, wheat germ, milk, eggs, cheese, fish	Coenzyme; part of 2 cellular reactions that make energy in cells called glycolysis and citric acid cycle	Itching and tingling	Painful tongue, chapped lips, cracks or sores at the corners of the mouth
B3 Niacin • Avocados, green peas, mushrooms, peanuts, tuna	Coenzyme; part of 2 cellular reactions that make energy in cells called glycolysis and citric acid cycle	Itching, burning, expansion of blood vessels (vasodilation)	Known as pellagra and referred to as the "3Ds": sun-sensitive dermatitis, diarrhea, and dementia; untreated leads to 4th D: death

Vitamin *Alternate Name* • *Food Sources*	*Importance*	*Effects of Excessiveness*	*Effects of Deficiency*
B5 Pantothenic acid • Almost all plant and animal foods	Precursor in synthesis of coenzyme A; essential for growth	None reported	Rare except in severe malnutrition; numbness and burning of hands and feet, headache, fatigue
B6 Pyridoxine • Beef liver, fish, fruit (other than citrus), potatoes	Coenzyme in amino acid and fat metabolism	Nerve damage, light sensitivity, nausea, heartburn	Microcytic (small cell) anemia, swollen tongue, cracks at the corners of the lips, depression, confusion, depressed immune function
B7 Biotin • Egg yolks, nuts and seeds, sweet potatoes	Coenzyme in many pathways	Increased urinating, abnormal sweating	Hair loss, red scaly face rash, depression, tingling and numbness of extremities
B9 Folate/folic acid • Leafy green vegetables, citrus fruits, beans, rice	Coenzyme in amino acid and nucleic acid metabolism	Anemia; in pregnant women there is an increased risk of spina bifida (neural tube birth defect)	Can mask vitamin B12 deficiency; nausea
B12 Cobalamin • Found naturally in animal products; meat, fish, eggs, milk products	Coenzyme in nucleic acid metabolism	Pernicious anemia	Bloating and diarrhea
C Ascorbic acid • Citrus fruit, broccoli, tomatoes	Coenzyme in many metabolic pathways	Kidney stones	Scurvy (rare), fatigue, impaired wound healing

Vitamin B3 (Niacin)

Clinical nutrition is the study of the relationship between diet and disease, oftentimes identifying absent nutrients that lead to disorders. One such disorder resulting from nutritional deficiency, specifically niacin, is pellagra. The term *pellagra* is derived from the Italian words, *pelle* for skin and *agra* for rough, referring to the skin inflammation and roughness characteristic of the disease. It is known as the "disease of the four D's" because of its resultant *d*iarrhea, *d*ermatitis (skin inflammation), *d*ementia, and *d*eath. Although it is rare in developed countries, it plagued the United States from 1906 to 1940. During this time, three million Americans were affected, and 100,000 people died of the disease. It was especially problematic in poor areas of the southern United States where meals were mainly *m*eat (pork fatback), *m*olasses, and *m*eal (cornmeal). Hence, it was dubbed the "3 M Diet."

The physician credited with linking poor diet with pellagra was Dr. Joseph Goldberger, who observed that malnourished people in orphanages, mental hospitals, and prisons developed the disease. At that time, it was assumed that germs caused the disease, not a nutritional deficiency. Dr. Goldberger, who wasn't the most ethical of practitioners, had a hunch that it might not be a germ-induced disorder. His 1915 experiments were conducted on Mississippi prisoners, who "volunteered" in exchange for sentence pardoning. Goldberger fed prisoners a very poor diet, which he believed was the cause of the pellagra. Within months, these "volunteers" did indeed develop pellagra. Later, a diet that included meat, fresh vegetables, and milk was introduced to the prison volunteers. Within a short period of time, the signs and symptoms of pellagra were reversed. The actual deficient nutrient causing the disease, niacin, wasn't discovered until 1937, which was eight years after Goldberger died from kidney cancer.

This story also brings up an important point about informed consent and using human subjects to conduct medical research. Today, in order for scientists to conduct studies on people, real volunteers must go through a rigorous process that is much more than voluntarily agreeing to participate in research. The person must fully understand the purpose of the research and its risks, scientists must adhere to ethical codes and regulations for using human subjects, and an institutional review board oversees the project—before and during. Moreover, when human subjects are involved, volunteers may disengage from the study at any time. This is important to note because history is replete with unethical research undertakings, notably the 1932 "Tuskegee Study of Untreated Syphilis in the Negro Male," an ethically unjustified research project undertaken by the United States Public Health Service. This study involved 600 black men, 399 with syphilis. It was undertaken to see what would happen to these men if the disease was not treated with antibiotics, which were known to cure the disease. The men had been misled and they thought they were being treated for "bad blood," a colloquial term for syphilis, anemia, and fatigue. Sadly, this study went on for 40 years.

In 1973 a class-action lawsuit was filed, and in 1974 a $10 million out-of-court settlement was reached. In this settlement, the U.S. government established the Tuskegee Health Benefit Program (THBP) to pay lifetime medical and burial expenses for all living participants. In 1975, wives, widows, and offspring were added. In 1995, health benefits were added. In 2004, the last study participant died; in 2009, the last widow died; currently there are 11 offspring receiving benefits.

Looking back at the water-soluble vitamins table, you'll note that peanuts are listed as a good source of niacin. In fact, nuts in general pack a nutritious punch as they are an excellent source of various vitamins and minerals. A 2019 study published in *Circulation*, found that the more nuts volunteers with type 2 diabetes ate, the less likely they were to die during the study and the less prone to heart disease they became. Okay, you're probably thinking, well, I'll just eat nuts and never die. Sounds good, but we still can't live forever. And remember that you need *all* the nutrients, and nuts don't contain every nutrient. What they did find was that people who ate five servings (one serving = one ounce) a week of almonds, pecans, pistachios, or walnuts were 34 percent less likely to die from cardiovascular causes than those people who ate less than one serving per month.

Are there heart-healthy benefits for nut eaters who don't have type 2 diabetes? Yes! A 2017 epidemiological study published in *Journal of the American College of Cardiology* found that people who ate an ounce of nuts several times a week were less likely to be diagnosed with heart disease. Compared to non-nut eaters, people who ate an ounce of nuts at least five times per week had a 20 percent lower risk of coronary heart disease. Epidemiological evidence found that both peanuts and tree nuts are heart healthy. Walnuts seemed to have the strongest effect, but almonds, cashews, and pistachios were also associated with reduced coronary artery disease. Peanut butter, however, doesn't confer those benefits, likely due to its processing, showing that whole food is better. Nuts are also rich in protein, fiber, and unsaturated fatty acids—more nutritional bang for the buck!

Vitamin B12 (Cobalamin)

Vitamin B12 is another essential vitamin; it's also known as cobalamin because it incorporates an ion of cobalt into its molecular structure.

It is also an interesting vitamin because of its association with a glyco-protein that is necessary for its absorption. This glycoprotein, which is secreted by stomach cells, is called intrinsic factor. In order for vitamin B12 to be absorbed, intrinsic factor attaches to it and carries it to the small intestines where it can be absorbed by blood vessels. The relation-ship between vitamin B12 and intrinsic factor is crucial because vitamin B12 plays an important role in cellular metabolism, forming red blood cells, making fatty acids and amino acids, and repairing DNA. If intrin-sic factor or vitamin B12 is absent, it leads to pernicious anemia, a con-dition whose main symptom is tiredness. Other signs and symptoms include pale skin, hand and feet numbness, shortness of breath, and confusion. Strict vegans are at risk of developing vitamin B12 deficiency because the vitamin can only be obtained from eating animals (meat) or animal products (milk and eggs). So it is important that vegans eat food fortified with vitamin B12 or take a supplement. Now's a good time to discuss the difference between fortified foods and enriched foods given the previous sentence. Fortified means that vitamins and/or min-erals that weren't originally found in that food have been added; an example is adding vitamin D to milk to enhance calcium absorption. Enriched means that vitamins and/or minerals that were lost during food processing have been added back; an example is adding vitamins lost during wheat processing to make enriched white flour. Vitamin B12 cannot be artificially made in the lab, so all sources—whether in forti-fied food or vitamin supplements—are derived from animals.

Under what circumstances might a person lack intrinsic factor? Lack of intrinsic factor results from autoimmune attack on the stom-ach's native parietal cells that make intrinsic factor, or it results if all or part of the stomach has been surgically removed. In those cases, vitamin B12 injections are necessary.

From an evolutionary perspective, it doesn't make much sense that if humans were herbivores, why would we require eating animals for this essential vitamin? It's a good question and can best be answered noting that evolution is not a straight path. It is a long and winding road. For mil-lions of years, we and our herbivore ancestors thrived on plants, so at one time in our history, we or the bacteria in our gut, likely made this essential vitamin. If we look at vegetarian mammals—who also need vitamin B12—bacteria in their large intestines produce vitamin B12. It's a nice symbiotic relationship. If we look at bacteria in our large intestine, they also produce vitamin B12. The difference, however, is *where* vitamin B12 is absorbed. In animals other than humans, vitamin B12 is absorbed in the *large* intestine;

in humans, we absorb vitamin B12 in the *small* intestine, with help from intrinsic factor. Thus, our bacteria produce it, but it winds up in our feces. At some point in our history when our ancestors began experimenting with eating animals, our small intestine must have begun absorbing the nutrient. If you recall from Chapter 2, nearly all nutrients are absorbed across the small intestines, not the large intestines.

Vitamin C (Ascorbic Acid)

A classic single-nutrient deficiency example comes from a step back in time and involves sailors. During the Age of Sail (1571–1862), approximately 50 percent of sailors died of a condition known as scurvy, a disease characterized by gum ulceration, tooth loss, and poor wound healing. It was caused by a diet lacking vitamin C. While life as a sailor was a horrific experience, scurvy was just as dreaded. Much has been written in the history of science about the link between scurvy and vitamin C deficiency and its story is interesting. Equally interesting is the fact that humans, guinea pigs, fruit bats, and some other simians (apes and monkeys) are the only mammals that cannot make their own vitamin C; thus, it must be obtained in the diet. Scurvy is rarely—if ever—seen in developed countries.

Taking a closer look at vitamin C, it is an essential vitamin. In nearly all aspects of life, essential means we need it, but when it comes to nutrition, essential means we have to obtain it from our diets because we don't make it ourselves. What happened that my dog and cat can make vitamin C, but I cannot? Somewhere along our evolution we experienced a genetic mutation affecting vitamin C. The gene for vitamin C synthesis still exists in our genome, can be identified, but it no longer functions. We know that his gene codes for the enzyme, L-gulonolactone oxidase, which is key to vitamin C synthesis. Our population wasn't wiped out as a result of no longer being able to synthesize vitamin C, because most primates of the time lived in an area rich with vitamin C infused citrus fruits, which they were already eating.

If scientists had a favorite vitamin, then vitamin C belongs to Linus Pauling (1901–1994). Linus Pauling was a scientist and humanitarian who received not one, but two unshared Nobel Prizes—for Chemistry (1954) and for Peace (1962). Receiving one Nobel Prize is a monumental achievement, but two is off the charts. Only three other people in the history of Nobel Prize awards have won the prize twice: Frederick Sanger (1958 and 1980), John Bardeen (1956 and 1972), and Marie Curie (1903 and 1911). Pauling is the only person to win it twice as a solo act. He published over 1,065 works from scientific papers and reviews to textbooks and popular books.

Pauling's popular books dealt with his vitamin C fascination. Two of those books are (1) *Vitamin C, the Common Cold and the Flu* and (2) *Cancer and Vitamin C*. At the time of their writing, they were viewed by the scientific community as quackery. Yet, they were both best sellers. Was Pauling onto something?

The common cold is one of the most common ailments affecting us. So it's very likely that you've heard that you should take vitamin C for a cold. But does vitamin C actually do anything for the common cold? Apparently, it does. Well, maybe it does. In a 1972 study, subjects who took 1,000 mg of vitamin C every day and who increased their dosage to 4,000 mg of vitamin C when they felt like they were coming down with a cold reduced their cold frequency by 9 percent and their number of sick days 14 percent. A review of the literature conducted in 2004 showed that vitamin C supplementation didn't prevent colds, but it could shorten the duration and severity of symptoms.

More recent studies show vitamin C to be a rock star. A 2017 study showed that vitamin C boosted the immune response. While another meta-analysis of non-randomized controlled trials published in 2018 demonstrated that if you already take vitamin C supplements and you get a cold, vitamin C supplementation may be beneficial. Yet, another published study analyzed 45 studies overall, 31 of which were randomized, and concluded that vitamin C consumption does not prevent the incidence of the common cold. Data conflict.

So what is a person supposed to do? There are over a couple hundred different viruses that cause the common cold and every person's immune response is difference. Maybe vitamin C would work against one of the strains affecting you. It might be worth a try. Since vitamin C is a water-soluble vitamin, it is probably best not to take an increased dosage all at once, but rather throughout the day so that the vitamin stays in you and isn't excreted in your urine. Nobody said nutrition science was easy.

Another area of keen research interest is the relationship between vitamin C consumption and cancer. Animal studies on mice have shown that vitamin C may protect against leukemia—a type of white blood cell cancer. If vitamin C levels drop, stem cells, which form the various types of blood cells may transform into abnormal leukemia cells. The research has been conducted *in vitro*, which means in a test tube, but not *in vivo*, which means in living organisms. Stay tuned as more research becomes available.

Fat-Soluble Vitamins

The fat-soluble vitamins include vitamin A (retinol), vitamin D (cholecalciferol), vitamin E (tocopherol), and vitamin K. As their name suggests, fat-soluble vitamins require fat solvents to dissolve. Each one of these, however, is needed to ensure good health. The amounts vary depending on age, but the important thing to note is that these are micronutrients, which means we need them in small amounts. They are so small that they are measured in milligrams or micrograms. If you're not familiar with the metric system, these amounts are teeny tiny! One milligram (mg) is equal to 0.000035 ounces (oz) and one microgram = 0.000000035 ounces. The best way to obtain these nutrients is to eat actual food. In fact, supplementing is not necessary if your diet is adequate. Yet, you've seen the nutritional supplements aisle at the grocery store: the shelves are stocked with vitamins.

Fat-soluble vitamins can accumulate in the body because they are not washed out as readily as water-soluble vitamins. If you've ever been around infants who are being introduced to solid foods, this can be easily apparent when foods rich in beta carotene, such as carrots and sweet potatoes, are added to the diet. Beta-carotene is a yellow-orange plant pigment and is a precursor of vitamin A. A precursor is a substance from which another is formed. Think of it as the forerunner. Some infants and children develop carotenemia, marked by yellow-orange skin particularly on the nose and cheeks, due to the increased levels of beta-carotene in the blood. It can also be seen in vegetarians.

A chart of the fat-soluble vitamins and alternate names, listing their importance, food sources, and the effects of excessiveness and deficiency is given below.

Fat-Soluble Vitamins Chart

Vitamin *Alternate Name* • *Food Sources*	*Importance*	*Effects of Excessiveness*	*Effects of Deficiency*
A Retinol • Eggs, fruits, vegetables	Necessary to produce visual pigments that absorb light, supports immune system	Liver damage, nausea	Night blindness; impaired growth, susceptibility to infections

Vitamin Alternate Name • Food Sources	Importance	Effects of Excessiveness	Effects of Deficiency
D Cholecalciferol • Fatty fish, cheese, egg yolks	Promotes proper use of calcium and phosphorus; bone growth, tooth development	Improper bone mineralization: rickets (in children), osteomalacia (in adults)	Calcium buildup in blood, nausea, vomiting
E Tocopherol • Vegetable oils, nuts, sunflower seeds, green leafy vegetables	Prevents breakdown of vitamin A and fatty acids	Nausea, diarrhea, headache	Disorientation and vision problems; muscle problems
K • Green leafy vegetables, broccoli, fish, eggs	Essential for formation of blood clotting factors	Liver dysfunction, jaundice; excessive blood clots	Bruising, excessive bleeding

Vitamin D, Calcium and Osteoporosis

Examples abound linking fat-soluble vitamin deficiency with disease, but a well-known one is linked to bone development. Rickets is a bone disease caused by vitamin D deficiency, which leads to bone softening and bowed legs in children. Vitamin D is necessary for calcium absorption. That means that in order for calcium to make its way into our bones, we need vitamin D to get it there. It doesn't end with skeletal deformity, though. Hypocalcemia—the medical term for low levels of calcium in the blood—can cause sustained muscle contractions (tetany), irritability, and bone fractures.

If there is one vitamin that is receiving a lot of hype right now, it is vitamin D, which was discovered in 1920. If vitamin D were discovered today, it likely would be considered a hormone on account of its behavior in the body. Not only do we get it from food, but we also make it. Let's break this down. There are actually two kinds of vitamin D: vitamin D2 and vitamin D3. Both types occur naturally in some foods like tuna and egg yolks. Other foods like milk, orange juice, and cereal are fortified with vitamin D2 and vitamin D3. Manufacturers add vitamin D because we generally can't get enough from food alone, and since 1930 it has been added to food to help reduce rickets. But our skin also makes vitamin D when it is exposed to sunlight. Through a series of biochemical reactions, when ultraviolet radiation (specifically UVB) hits our skin, cholesterol in our skin cells (remember from previous chapters that cholesterol makes up portions of our cell membranes) is converted to vitamin D3 by our liver and kidneys. As a fat-soluble vitamin, we store what we don't use in our fat cells. When our body needs vitamin D—and it doesn't matter whether it is vitamin D from food or vitamin D from sunlight—the liver and kidneys convert the stored vitamin D into calcitriol. Calcitriol is the active form of vitamin D that the body "knows" how to use. Calcitriol is prescribed medically to treat osteoporosis, and it is given to people with chronic kidney disease who are unable to manufacture it. Osteoporosis is a medical condition in which the bones become brittle and fragile as a result of bone tissue loss. The weakened bone tissue increases the risk of fractures. Look at Figure 7.1 to see the appearance of a femur (thigh bone) that has normal bone tissue compared to a femur with osteoporotic bone. Sunscreens, gray days, and darker skin can limit vitamin D production, so it's always wise to find some food that contains vitamin D to eat.

Low blood vitamin D levels has been linked to seasonal affective disorder (SAD) and depression. SAD is a form of depression that occurs during late autumn and winter and is thought to be caused by diminished amounts of sunlight. In a 2015 study, researchers found an association between vitamin D levels and depression in otherwise healthy young adult women. Again, if a person chooses to supplement with vitamin D, blood tests should be done and evaluated by healthcare professionals.

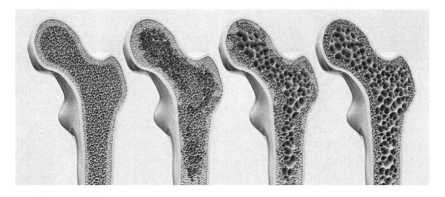

Figure 7.1 The progression of osteoporosis. The bone on the far left is a normal thigh bone (femur) with healthy internal architecture. The bone on the far right is a thigh bone with osteoporosis. Note how the density of the internal bone architecture changes, becoming much more brittle and open in the osteoporotic bone (from Shutterstock).

There are additional benefits to getting vitamin D from sunlight: being outdoors is really good for us. There are other health benefits that come from spending about 20 minutes in the great outdoors, enjoying Mother Nature. Being outside may boost your energy as much as one cup of caffeinated coffee. Natural sunlight diminishes stress. It also mitigates pain, decreasing the need for pain medication. A dose of Mother Nature also helps with seasonal affective disorder, even if it's a cold, damp, dreary day. The outdoors boosts our creativity, restores focus, and connects us to the natural world. It's all good!

What about vitamin D and prostate cancer? The male prostate has numerous vitamin D receptors, which convert inactive vitamin D into active vitamin D. Some research has shown that when men take more than 2,000 mg of calcium per day from supplements, there is an increased risk of prostate cancer. It might not be the calcium that is at fault; it might be a lack of active vitamin D. Again, more research is needed.

As I write, the coronavirus has claimed more than 642,000 lives in the United States. By the time this book is published, that number is projected to be much higher. We know that inadequate levels of vitamin D are associated with hypertension, diabetes, cardiovascular disease, and metabolic syndrome. When one of these conditions exists within a person who has contracted coronavirus infection, comorbidity results. To that end, very recent research has shown that adequate vitamin D levels are protective against COVID-19 complications and mortality. Other research has shown that vitamin D may regulate the immune system and also reduce inflammation. Low levels of vitamin D appear to increase the risk of coronavirus infection. Identifying just how much vitamin D you need is a bit tricky. Some people need 2,000 IUs while others need 4,000 IUs, and the only way to know what your appropriate level is requires a blood test for 25 hydroxy vitamin D. Given the health benefits of having adequate vitamin D levels, the test might be worth getting, especially if you are unable to get outdoors for natural vitamin D synthesis from sunshine or if your diet lacks adequate amounts of vitamin D.

Taking a combination of 400 IU vitamin D and 500 mg calcium twice per day may reduce the risk of getting benign paroxysmal positional vertigo (BPPV). BPPV is the sudden sensation that you are spinning and people who suffer from this condition experience brief episodes of mild dizziness to intense dizziness. It can be quite debilitating. Researchers found that supplementation with vitamin D and calcium should be considered to prevent vertigo from recurring in patients with frequent attacks of BPPV, especially when blood vitamin D level is below normal.

Remember that bone is living tissue that is capable of growth. This is called bone turnover and refers to building bone density. Two types of cells are involved: osteoclasts and osteoblasts. As osteoclasts break down bone, osteoblasts build up bone. To help you remember which cell does what, osteoclast is derived from the word parts *osteo* meaning *bone* and *klastes* meaning *breaker*. *Osteoblast* comes from the word part *osteo* meaning *bone* plus *-blast* meaning a cell that *builds*. The goal is for osteoblasts to either outpace osteoclasts or to stay even with them. It's also important to note that during adulthood, bone *length* will not be affected by exercise because the *epiphyseal plates*, otherwise known as *growth plates*, have ossified (fused), thereby preventing long bone growth. This means that bones can grow thicker, but not longer.

There's quite a relationship between calcium and vitamin D. We know that in order for calcium to be absorbed across the intestines, vitamin D is necessary. Calcium circulating within the bloodstream is necessary for neuromuscular and heart functions. Because it is vital to our survival, our body doesn't allow blood calcium levels to drop. It does this through a process of negative feedback: If blood calcium level decreases, parathyroid hormone is released. Parathyroid hormone comes from four tiny glands embedded on the posterior (back) surface of your thyroid gland in your neck. This hormone mobilizes calcium from bones. Basically, it causes bone tissue to break down to release its calcium into the bloodstream so that nerves, muscles, and the heart function like they should. However, if the bones are being robbed of their calcium, then they become weaker and by extension, are more prone to break. While we know that vitamin D deficiency increases the risk of osteoporosis and bone fractures, we still don't have good data on how much vitamin D and/or calcium should be used in supplements. Diets containing foods rich in vitamin D and calcium are always best.

Time to interject a little more physiology science here. Blood tests that measure calcium levels are no indication for bone health. Because of the aforementioned negative feedback—when one thing is high, something else will kick in to bring it down—the bloodstream will always be the first to get the calcium to maintain vital functioning of our organs. In our body, it works like this: If blood calcium level drops, parathyroid hormone (PTH) is released from the parathyroid glands. This hormone causes osteoclasts to break down bone and release its calcium to the blood. If blood calcium is adequate or high, another hormone called *calcitonin* from the thyroid gland delivers the calcium to osteoblasts that use it to build bone. It's a delicate interplay among circulating levels of blood calcium, intact bone tissue, and circulating hormones. Here's a quick scenario:

Hypocalcemia (low blood calcium) → parathyroid hormone from parathyroid glands is released → osteoclasts break down bone → calcium released into bloodstream → other organs use calcium
   Goal: to increase blood calcium level

Hypercalcemia (high blood calcium) → calcitonin from thyroid gland is released → calcium delivered to osteoblasts → bone is built
   Goal: to decrease blood calcium level

Bone density is measured using an instrument called a densitometer. It measures the photographic density—or degree of darkness—of an image on a film or photographic print when a light source is aimed at a structure. In a clinical setting, dual-energy x-ray absorptiometry (DEXA) measures bone mineral density using two x-ray beams with different energy levels that are aimed at the person's bones. Soft tissues also absorb light, but when soft tissue absorption is subtracted out, bone density is determined from the absorption of each beam by the bone. It is an excellent tool for evaluating osteoporosis.

Osteoporosis has sometimes been referred to as a "pediatric problem with geriatric consequences." The reason is because bone mass peaks during the third decade of life; thereafter, we begin to lose bone. However, weight-bearing exercises throughout life can do much to thwart bone loss. As a disorder, osteoporosis risk is rooted in human evolution. Early humans living along equatorial regions had diets with abundant calcium and vitamin D. Calcium was consumed in food while vitamin D was made by the skin exposed to sunlight. As humans migrated out of equatorial regions to higher latitudes and adopted agricultural practices, vitamin D synthesis was diminished and calcium content in food was reduced. If we look at modern day hunter-gatherer humans still living in Africa, South America, and New Guinea, they still have diets very high in calcium. And the calcium is not coming from dairy products. Calcium-rich foods consumed are leafy greens, nuts, roots, and tubers.

In addition to diet, weight-bearing exercise is important for treating and preventing osteoporosis. Muscles are attached to bones and both are living tissues. As such, because exercise stresses tissues, growth is stimulated, resulting in increased muscle mass and increased bone density. Weight-bearing exercises, such as lifting weights, climbing stairs, walking, and jogging, are those that force you to work against gravity and are best for maintaining muscle and bone. Swimming and bicycling are good exercises for cardiovascular benefits but are not considered weight-bearing. Exercise also has added benefits like increasing strength, coordination, and balance. These in turn can help prevent falls and related fractures and improve mobility, which leads to independence and greater health.

Supplementation may also help prevent osteoporosis. Hormonal changes, calcium deficiency, and vitamin D deficiency can lead to osteoporosis, however, determining the correct dosage of vitamin D is difficult. Recent research is indicating that the only people who experience real benefits from vitamin D supplementation are those who are already vitamin D deficient.

Other studies have shown that taking vitamin D supplements to prevent osteoporosis is not borne out in the literature. In a 2019 study published in *JAMA*, researchers studied 311 people without osteoporosis who were between 55 and 70 years old. The randomized, controlled study was conducted over three years. Researchers divided the participants into three groups and gave one group 400 IU (former RDA), another 4,000 IU, and the third group received 10,000 IU (the upper tolerable limit). IU stands for international units and is the standard used for measuring this vitamin. Researchers measured bone mineral density at the beginning and end of the study. Their findings showed that in people taking 10,000 IU, bone mineral density in the tibia (shin bone) actually dropped, while those taking 4,000 IU showed decreased bone mineral density in the radius (arm bone running from the elbow to the wrist), and there were no differences in bone strength among the groups. One study subject developed calcium in the urine. This means that scientific findings do not support any benefit of high-dose vitamin D supplementation for bone health.

Genetic differences may also account for our varying responses to vitamin D supplementation. Studies on type 2 diabetic patients showed that vitamin D metabolic-related genes may affect blood levels of vitamin D when given vitamin D3 supplements.

Science is an ongoing endeavor. To date, researchers still are showing that for the most part, supplements are not improving health except in people who are deficient. While low vitamin D levels may be associated with disease, supplements don't seem to prevent them. In a 2019 meta-analysis published in *JAMA Cardiology*, findings did not support taking vitamin D supplements for heart disease. Meta-analyses are good to review because these types of studies examine data from a large number of independent studies done on the same subject and use statistical analysis to determine overall trends. These types of studies are robust because they can analyze findings across thousands of subjects among scientific peer-reviewed papers.

Vitamin K

Vitamin K is actually a group of vitamins, such as K_1 (phylloquinone), K_2 (menaquinone), and K_3 (menadione) that play a role in blood clotting by synthesizing certain proteins—blood clotting factors—needed for coagulation. The "K" in vitamin K comes from the Danish word *Koagulation*. Vitamin K is found mainly in green leafy vegetables, and vitamin K_1 is found in the highest amounts in such plants. Demonstrating another symbiotic relationship, bacteria in our gut convert K_1 to K_2. Bacteria are also able to synthesize vitamin K_2 in the absence of vitamin K_1.

People who take blood thinners (anti-coagulants), such as warfarin and coumarin, limit their intake of foods containing vitamin K. Conversely, vitamin K is the antidote for anti-coagulant overdose. Newborns are given a prophylactic intramuscular injection of vitamin K at birth because their clotting factors are 30 percent–60 percent that of an adult. The diminished clotting factors at birth are likely due to the sterility of their intestines or at least low bacterial count in the intestines.

Major Body Minerals

Time to discuss the major minerals of the body. The body's major minerals along with their symbols are calcium (Ca), chloride (Cl), magnesium (Mg), phosphorus (P), potassium (K), and sodium (Na). Refer back to the chart at the beginning of the chapter if you'd like an accounting of all the major minerals. As you likely noticed, the abbreviations for potassium and sodium might not make a lot of sense. This is where knowing word derivations comes in handy.

Potassium is a synonym for kalium, derived from the word *quali*, which means *potash*. Okay, you likely see *kalium* and *K*, but potash is another quandary. Potassium is an alkaline metallic element and potash is an alkaline potassium compound. Potassium occurs abundantly in nature in combinations such as potassium acetate, potassium carbonate, and potassium hydroxide. Its salts are used medicinally. Salts are compounds formed by the interaction of an acid (anything with a pH less than 7) and a base (anything with a pH greater than 7). Proto-typical salts are sodium chloride (NaCl) and potassium chloride (KCl). Sodium chloride is common table salt. Potassium chloride is also commonly used as a salt substitute, meaning sodium has been replaced with potassium. Low-salt diets frequently use potassium chloride instead of sodium chloride. Our bodies require the ionic form of each: K^+, Na^+, and Cl^-. As you've heard, opposites attract, so both potassium and sodium, which have a positive charge (+) are attracted to chloride, which has a negative charge, (−). So we get KCl for potassium chloride and NaCl for sodium chloride. We have fairly equal amounts of sodium and chloride in our body.

Sodium is a synonym for natrium, derived from the word *natrum*. It is a metallic element and its salts are used extensively in medicine and industry. Sodium ions are the most abundant extracellular (*extra* = outside + *cellular* = cells) ions in the body. Our cells are bathed in fluid called *extracellular fluid* and sodium ions are the most populous of all the ions found there. This makes sense because ions have many roles in cellular functions. Thus, the major minerals are the ions in the body.

For the sake of simplicity, think of ions as electrolytes—the same stuff found in the sports drink, Gatorade. Sodium and chloride ions are important for regulating the osmotic concentration of our body fluids. Stick with me here; this is important. Osmotic concentration is crucial for equalizing concentrations on each side of cell membranes. Think of it this way: We have trillions of cells in our bodies. These cells are more or less circular in shape. Forming the shape is a membrane. Remember that phospholipids and cholesterol were important to helping form cell membranes. Inside the cell membrane are all the working parts of cells called organelles, each with a specific function. Outside the cell membrane is the watery fluid in which our cells are surrounded. This membrane allows the passage of some substances but restricts the passage of others. Cells are very particular. Mineral ions—those electrolytes—buffer our body fluids, ensuring that various fluids are kept at the appropriate pH—not too acidic and not too basic, but just right depending on what that body fluid is. Those fluids could be blood, extracellular fluid, or the special fluid called cerebrospinal fluid that bathes the brain and spinal cord. Minerals, like vitamins, are also important as cofactors that work with enzymes. It's like having a colleague helping you do your job. You often see these minerals listed on food labels. Here is a chart of the body's major minerals, their importance, the effects of too many, and the effects of not enough.

Major Body Minerals Chart

Mineral	Importance	Effects of Excessiveness	Effects of Deficiency
Calcium	Needed for neuron and muscle function and building bones and teeth	Kidney stones	Osteoporosis
Chloride	Needed for forming hydrochloric acid (HCl)	Affects mineral balance; dehydration	Irregular heartbeat
Magnesium	Cofactor of enzymes	Irregular heartbeat, confusion, low blood pressure	Muscle spasms, nausea, fatigue
Phosphorus	Needed to make nucleic acids and to build bones and teeth	Muscle spasms	Muscle weakness
Potassium	Needed for cellular membrane functions, cofactor of enzymes	Irregular heartbeat	Irregular heartbeat
Sodium	Needed for cellular membrane functions, cofactor of enzymes	Increased blood pressure	Hyponatremia (low salt in the blood); muscle weakness, muscle cramps, seizure, coma

Trace Body Minerals

Trace minerals are essential food factors required in only small quantities in the body. The trace minerals include cobalt, copper, fluoride, iodine, iron, manganese, selenium, and zinc.

Have you ever wondered why table salt contains the trace mineral iodine? By itself, salt is just sodium and chloride. However, iodized salt is ordinary table salt with added iodine. Iodine is an element that is necessary for normal thyroid function. In lesser developed countries, iodine deficiency is a major public health problem. Iodine is found naturally in food grown near seacoasts but occurs in lesser amounts or not at all in food grown in other areas. So, if vegetables are grown in iodine-deficient soils, iodine cannot be taken up by the plant's root system, and thus the vegetables do not contain iodine. Superficially this doesn't sound too problematic, but iodine-deficient diets lead to goiter (a huge lump on the neck caused by thyroid gland enlargement), neuro-cognitive impairment, and hypothyroidism.

As a crucial micronutrient that we must get from food (our bodies cannot make it), it has been added to table salt as potassium iodide since 1924. Circle back to the neurocognitive impairment: adding iodine to salt actually boosted Americans' IQ scores. Intelligence data between 1921 and 1927 were evaluated and it was found that adding iodine to the diet had mental benefits. Nowadays, we get plenty of iodized salt in our diets and iodine deficiency in America has been relegated to the history books.

Salt

Common table salt is a topic of many health debates. For years, cardiologists have touted it to be the culprit for high blood pressure. Then, new research suggested that if the kidneys are doing their jobs, it really shouldn't matter how much salt you consume because the excess would be excreted in the urine. Other research stated that people who are *salt sensitive* should limit their intake because their kidneys retained the salt. Now, research is showing a link between salt and increased risk of stroke and cognitive impairment, irrespective of high blood pressure.

Books have been written about salt and human health. We'll keep it simple here: According to the World Health Organization (WHO), most people consume too much salt, which is around nine to 12 grams per day. The recommended level is less than five grams per day. The WHO estimates that lowering salt consumption could prevent about 2.5 million deaths worldwide annually.

Is there a difference between sea salt and kosher salt? There are obvious differences if you compare sea salt, kosher salt, and table salt. Sea salt and kosher salt have bigger, coarser crystals than table salt. Sea salt is made by evaporating seawater so it may have some trace minerals that give some sea salts various colors. Kosher salt is made from salt crystals and is usually not iodized. Sea salt and kosher salt are used in cooking to enhance flavor, but like table salt, intake should be monitored because too much has negative health consequences. It's interesting to note that kosher salt really has nothing to do with Jewish dietary law. The reference to kosher salt dates back to around the 1920s when coarse-grained salt was used to absorb blood from meat that was prepared according to the requirements of Jewish dietary law.

Kosher foods are those prepared according to Jewish dietary law derived from the books of Leviticus and Deuteronomy. As such, animals must be slaughtered and prepared in a particular way. According to Jewish law, kosher meats are derived from animals whose blood has been drained at slaughter. Jewish dietary law also forbids eating pigs and shellfish, meat and milk cannot be cooked or consumed together, and separate utensils must be kept and used for each.

There also seems to be a gut-brain axis, a so-called communication venue between our gastrointestinal tract and our brains, which is influenced by dietary salt. High salt intake may cause immune changes in the gut, resulting in increased vulnerability of the brain to an attack by native immune cells. When native immune cells mistakenly attack its own body, we refer to this as an autoimmune disease. Although this research is in its infancy, it suggests that excessive salt consumption might negatively impact the brain—regardless of salt's effect on blood pressure.

The implications for reducing salt intake are broad because the newly identified gut-brain connection could be extended to other known autoimmune diseases. Examples include inflammatory bowel disease, multiple sclerosis, psoriasis, and rheumatoid arthritis. The gut-brain axis has also been implicated from a microbiome perspective as well, giving rise to the microbiota-gut-brain axis. The microbiome—the microscopic organisms that live in and on us—is a hot topic right now. It's hot because we're finding out more and more just how closely associated we are with those things we cannot see. The human genome is our full set of genetic instructions contained in our cells that makes us human, and we're learning that the microbiome may influence our personal genome. If you count all the cells in our body, we're about 43 percent human—the remaining cells make up our microbiome. The genes of our microbiome contain between two million and 20 million microbial genes. This second set of genes is being referred to as our second genome and our gut microorganisms are closely associated with various nervous, endocrine, and immune communications. While it seems to play a role in various diseases including Parkinson's disease, Alzheimer's disease, schizophrenia, inflammatory bowel disease, and multiple sclerosis, the microbiome also appears to influence whether cancer drugs work and may also be linked to depression and autism. Stay tuned as more research becomes available, and we learn more about promoting gut health through probiotics and prebiotics.

Iron

Iron is a nutritional mineral whose main purpose is to form part of the hemoglobin molecule in red blood cells. Hemoglobin carries oxygen throughout the body for use by our cells. Hemoglobin also helps remove carbon dioxide, which is a byproduct of cellular metabolism. Iron is also part of the oxygen-carrying protein, myoglobin, found in our muscles. Iron is needed for normal physical growth, neurological development, cellular functioning, and for synthesis of some hormones. It is found naturally in many foods, as an additive, or found in dietary supplements. When iron levels are low, a person feels weak and tired. If iron levels drop too low, iron-deficiency anemia, a condition in which there is red blood cell deficiency or hemoglobin deficiency, results. When this condition comes on slowly, the symptoms are vague; with time, the person becomes pale and extremely fatigued.

There are two types of dietary iron that we consume: heme and nonheme. In general, heme iron comes from animals and nonheme iron comes from plants. Meat contains both types of iron. The two types are molecularly different as heme iron has a porphyrin ring, which is a pigment, at the center of the molecule. In the body, heme iron has a higher bioavailability than does nonheme iron.

Food types can enhance or inhibit iron bioavailability. For example, vitamin C enhances nonheme iron absorption, but phytate (found in grains and beans) and some polyphenols inhibit nonheme iron absorption. Calcium might reduce bioavailability for both heme and nonheme iron. Iron bioavailability is about 14 percent–18 percent from mixed diets (containing both animal and plant heme) and 5 percent–12 percent from vegetarian diets. Food cooked in iron skillets also picks up the iron from the pan, enhancing iron amounts in the food.

While we know that we need iron for the ever-important oxygen-carrying proteins hemoglobin and myoglobin, its role in heart disease has been debated for years. The "iron hypothesis," first introduced in 1981 posited that the reason men had higher risk of coronary heart disease than women until menopause was due to menstruation: Basically, men had higher iron stores than women because menstruating women were slightly anemic during their lives due to blood loss through monthly periods. Then, when women stopped menstruating, their risk for coronary heart disease was level with men. Recent studies are now bolstering the link between red meat consumption and heart disease because there appears to be a strong association between heme iron and potentially deadly coronary heart disease. Future research is necessary to establish possible mechanisms.

Magnesium

Magnesium is a mineral found in spices, nuts, cereals, cocoa, and spinach. It's often confused with manganese because the spellings are similar. Most of the magnesium in the body is found in our bones and skeletal muscles. As a supplement, it is used to relieve nighttime muscle cramps, restless leg syndrome, and constipation; to increase vitamin D levels; and to help with insomnia. But do any of these have merit?

Beginning with muscle cramps, the research is showing that magnesium supplements probably don't prevent leg nighttime muscle cramps. There is limited evidence supporting the use of magnesium or vitamin B12 for nocturnal leg cramps. Furthermore, quinine, found in tonic water, is no longer recommended to treat leg cramps. Most leg cramps are due to nerve problems, not electrolyte abnormalities. Yet, magnesium bisglycinate chelate supplements at 300 mg/day did help pregnant women experiencing leg cramps.

Restless leg syndrome (RLS) is a disorder characterized by unpleasant tickling, twitching, or pain in the legs when sitting or lying down that is only relieved by moving them. The cause is unknown, although people with RLS often have kidney disease or iron deficiency. Prescription medication is available to treat the condition, but some people find relief from magnesium supplements. There are no well-done studies in the scientific literature supporting the use of magnesium for RLS.

Magnesium can be used to treat constipation. Recall the well-known over-the-counter laxative, Phillips' Milk of Magnesia (MOM)? Good ole MOM can treat constipation, upset stomach, and heartburn. Taking 300 mg magnesium supplements can also ease constipation. However, taking too much can cause diarrhea and people with kidney disorders should avoid magnesium supplements.

Magnesium plays a role in vitamin D activation, in turn regulating calcium and phosphorus balance, which are important to bone growth and maintenance. Enzymes that metabolize vitamin D, require magnesium as a cofactor. Therefore, vitamin D increases magnesium absorption and low magnesium levels make vitamin D ineffective.

Using magnesium for insomnia at a dosage of 400 mg/day may indirectly help insomnia. In a small study, people with mental and physical stress benefited from magnesium supplementation as the supplement reduced stress as measured by heart rate variability. This in turn might cause relaxation and improved ability to sleep.

That was our walk through the vitamins and minerals. The take-home message is that as best as we can, we should get all our nutrients from our diets instead of supplements. In some cases, it does make sense to use supplements, but for the most part taking them is not beneficial.

8

The Sustenance of Life

*Water, Fluid Balance
and the Environment*

Water

Found in all animal and vegetable tissues, water is the necessary ingredient for earthly life. We rely on that compound of hydrogen and oxygen with the chemical formula H_2O. Depending on our fat and protein reserves, we can live for quite some time without food, but water is a different story. Without water, we become dehydrated and suffer some pretty bad consequences within days. In fact, we will likely die within a week or so without water. Water has some interesting properties and is an excellent solvent that is able to dissolve more substances than any other liquid. It's also necessary for many biological functions.

In the body, fluid balance is achieved through a delicate relationship with electrolytes (minerals), for you also can't have fluid balance without electrolyte balance. These fluids are compartmentalized into semi-solid and liquid compartments. As such, we have a semi-solid compartment made up of mostly of proteins, followed by lipids, then minerals, and finally carbohydrates. As you can see, we truly are what we eat. The liquid compartments are the intracellular fluid and extracellular fluid, together accounting for 50 percent–60 percent of the total volume of water in the body. *Intracellular fluid* is the liquid found *within cells* that surrounds all the organelles, keeping them suspended in a jelly-like matrix. *Extracellular fluid*, found *around cells*, is made up of interstitial fluid of peripheral tissues and blood plasma of circulating blood. Fluids making up interstitial fluid include lymph (where immune cells called lymphocytes are found), aqueous humor (in our eyeballs), cerebrospinal fluid (surrounding the brain and spinal cord), perilymph and endolymph (in our inner ears), synovial fluid (around joints), and serous fluid (surrounding the lungs, hearts, and intestines). Here's a summary.

Semi-Solid Compartment
    Proteins
    Lipids
    Minerals
    Carbohydrates
Intracellular Fluid
    Inside cells
    Liquid surrounding cellular organelles
Extracellular fluid
    Outside cells
    Interstitial fluid
        Lymph
        Aqueous humor
        Cerebrospinal fluid
        Perilymph
        Endolymph
        Synovial fluid
        Serous fluid

Water has many roles throughout the body. For example, nutrients are carried throughout the body via blood, which is mostly water. Blood is made up of solids—mostly red blood cells—and liquid. The liquid part of blood is known as plasma, and water makes up 92 percent of that plasma. Other important jobs of water include serving as the solvent for vitamins, minerals (electrolytes), amino acids, and glucose. In the body, water balance implies electrolyte balance because you can't have one without the other. Water is the medium for biochemical reactions in the body; it bathes and lubricates our joints; and it helps with shock absorption between our spinal vertebrae. Another important feature of water is that it helps to maintain body temperature—think about sweating on a hot summer day. Water also makes up most our body weight. As you can see, it is vital to survival.

What are our main sources of water? Most of the water we have in our body comes from the water content of the food we eat and the liquids we drink. Maintaining water balance is critical to carrying out normal body functions: Too little water results in dehydration while too much can lead to water intoxication. It's a delicate balance.

The body always tries to strike a water balance, whereby the water we take in equals the amount lost through various routes. We lose water through breathing, sweating, urinating, and defecating. If you want to see water you lose through breathing, it's easy to do: On a cool day, sit in the car with the windows up. After a little while (the time is temperature dependent), you'll see condensation on the windows as a result of your breathing. Water balance ensures homeostasis—the body's internal balance—and sodium and potassium are two minerals that play important roles in achieving balance.

It's very likely you've heard that we should drink at least eight glasses of water per day. In fact, your own doctor may have even told you to do so. Today, it's nearly impossible to walk down the street without seeing a person with some sort of water bottle, chugging dutifully. Have you ever stopped to ask yourself "why?" What's magical about the number 8? The truth is, the eight-glass a day rule is a myth! It's a myth that dates back to 1945. In 1945, the Food and Nutrition Board of the National Research Council recommended that adults should consume about 2.5 liters of water a day, noting that most of it is already found in the food we eat. Yes, that's right: for whatever reason, the first part of that sentence stuck, i.e., "consume about 2.5 liters of water a day," while the second part of that sentence never made it to center stage. Let's do the math: 2.5 liters = about 85 ounces (84.5351, actually) → there are 8 ounces in a cup = 85 ounces/8 ounces = 10.625 cups. Well, 10.625 cups are *close* to eight cups. Close counts in horseshoes and apparently in conversion scales, too. Some circles even call this the 8 × 8 rule for eight, eight-ounce glasses of water.

To date, there is no scientific evidence supporting the notion that you should drink eight glasses of water per day. Yet, the myth persists. In reality, you get plenty of water just by eating and drinking normally. The healthy body already has systems in place to ensure you are not dehydrated. The scientific term for water regulation is osmoregulation, derived from the term *osmo* meaning water. Water balance is maintained through hormone regulation and thirst quenching, both of which involve our nervous and urinary systems. Our brains (nervous system) regulate water intake and our brains and kidneys (urinary system) regulate water output.

An important hormone for water regulation and the thirst mechanism is antidiuretic hormone (ADH). Antidiuretic hormone, also called *vasopressin*, does a good job of monitoring for dehydration. Breaking the word apart, *anti* means *against* while *diuretic* means *causing urination*, thus, ADH is secreted to prevent urination. Think of it this way:

ADH release = urine retention
No ADH = urination

Here's the lowdown: If body water levels begin to drop, ADH (vasopressin) will be released from a special area in the brain that signals the kidneys to retain water from the blood filtering through them. If the kidneys retain water, more water will stay in your bloodstream instead of becoming urine. This helps you to stay well hydrated.

The physiological mechanisms and neural regulation of thirst are complicated. If your body needs water, you get thirsty, and you drink. The more water you drink, the more water gets into your body. As we age, thirst sensitivity declines, so older people do have a greater risk of becoming dehydrated because ADH sensitivity decreases with age. For this reason, it's always good to check fluid intake in older folks. An easy assessment you can do any time to check your own water level is to pinch the skin on the back of your hand. Skin should be relatively elastic, like a rubber band. If the skin snaps back to its normal position quickly, your body's water level is fine. If it takes a few seconds to return to normal, it could be a sign of dehydration.

There are cases in which drinking 64 ounces (eight glasses) of water a day *are* warranted, however. For example, drinking this volume of water is advised to prevent kidney stones in people who are susceptible to kidney stone formation. If you've had a kidney stone in the past, you are susceptible to having a kidney stone in the future. So you'd be one of those people who should drink extra fluid, and water is the best fluid. Increased fluid intake is also advisable after strenuous exercise to replace fluid lost through sweating and heavy breathing.

Since we're made up of so much water, isn't water good for me, regardless of the source? Yes, water is good for us, but it's better to drink plain water rather than sugary sodas. But drinking too much water can be bad and it can happen, despite physiological mechanisms in place to prevent it. Too much water intake, known as *water intoxication*, occurs when water intake exceeds the kidneys' ability to excrete enough water. Basically, you can't urinate enough to get rid of the excess fluid. Water intoxication can happen if you drink too much water too quickly or too much fluid is infused too quickly through an IV. If this happens, fluid builds up, causing overhydration, which leads to brain swelling. Brain swelling can lead to death. In fact, in January 2007, water intoxication caused the death of a 28-year-old Sacramento, California, woman who was a contestant of an on-air KDND FM radio contest. The prize was a Nintendo Wii video console and the contest was called "Hold Your Wee for a Wii." Contestants were required to drink as much water as possible without urinating in order to win. This woman ended up dying a totally preventable death, had she only known.

Water intoxication can also occur in infants. Breast milk and infant formula provide babies with all the necessary fluids, so additional water is not necessary in healthy infants. Too much water dilutes a baby's normal sodium levels—wherever water goes, sodium follows—which can lead to seizures, coma, brain damage, and possible death.

Planetary Water

Water is vital to life, which is why 71 percent of the Earth's surface is covered in it. Of that 71 percent, about 96.5 percent is found in the oceans. We also get water from the air (water vapor), in rivers and lakes, in icecaps and glaciers, and in the ground as soil moisture and aquifers. While surface water is easily visualized, there is more water stored underground in aquifers. Regardless of the source, we need fresh, clean water to sustain life.

If so much of the planet is covered in seawater, can't we use that to sustain us? No, we can't drink seawater for our water needs because it contains too much salt. Like the infant example above, salt dilutes the water, so in addition to it tasting bad, drinking seawater would cause dehydration. If you did drink seawater, the salt would cause us to urinate more water than we drank, and we'd end up thirstier than when we started. While we do need the sodium and chloride that makes up salt for normal biological functions, we have systems in place to ensure balance. The concentration of salt in seawater is greater than our kidneys can process, and our kidneys can only make urine that is less salty than seawater. For these reasons, salt accumulates in the blood and we would eventually die of dehydration.

Some animals have adapted mechanisms that enable them to drink seawater. For example, very large oceanic birds such as the albatross have salt glands behind their eyes that excrete excess salt out through their beak tips. Other animals have evolutionary adaptations that allow them to conserve water. Kangaroo rats that live in the desert conserve water because their kidneys are able to excrete highly concentrated urine. This means that solutes are excreted with relatively little water in the urine. This happens to you as well: if you are dehydrated or on the verge of dehydration, the scant urine you excrete will be quite concentrated. You can note this by color: concentrated urine is dark while dilute urine is light. Camels are other animals that have evolved to survive low-to-no-water conditions as they are able to retain heat energy without adverse effects and can survive for a week in the desert without water.

Humans, on the other hand, can survive about 24 hours in the desert without water. In non-desert environments, a human can live about a week—give or take a few days—without water. We can live much longer without food. In fact, Indian nationalist, spiritual leader, and political activist Mahatma Gandhi survived 21 days without food. There is no hard and fast rule for how long a person can live without either because there are so many variables like age, activity level, overall health, and ambient environment, that figure into the dehydration equation.

Because water can be a scarce commodity, science technology is working on ways to desalinate seawater. Current techniques, such as desalination, are very energy intensive. One desalination technique in use today is reverse osmosis whereby water is pushed through a membrane that retains the salt and other particles but allows the water to pass through it. The retained particles create a brine. This process is used on ocean vessels and submarines.

Eighty percent of the fresh water on the planet is used to produce food and other agricultural products. The largest agricultural water footprints are found in the beef and dairy industries followed by poultry farming. Large concentrated animal feeding operations (CAFOs) were discussed in Chapter 6. However, when we discuss the environmental impact, there is no denying statistics. Mature cows drink from seven to 24 gallons of water per day, depending on the temperature, and active dairy cows drink about twice that amount. There is also indirect water to factor in. This is the amount of water used to grow the feed that the cows eat. Feed grain for animal consumption uses 56 percent of the total water consumed in the United States. To put it into perspective, it takes about 1,700 gallons of water to produce one pound of beef and 576 gallons for one pound of pork. For comparison, it takes 108 gallons of water to harvest one pound of corn. Of course, it only takes about 100 days to grow corn to maturity, while it takes about 995 days to grow cattle to maturity. The human to food animal ratio is an interesting figure:

There are about seven billion people on the planet and about 20 billion animals raised for food. This means that there are about 2.85 animals per human.

Another concern is the amount of antibiotics that make their way into our water supply. When animals live in close quarters to one another, antibiotics must be used to prevent and treat infection. It's a rule of nature that proximity breeds infection. Add to this the amount of antibiotics that people consume and then flush down the drain or the toilet. In the United States, an estimated 35,000 people die of an antibiotic-resistant infection while at least two million people get an antibiotic-resistance infection yearly. According to the CDC, antibiotic resistance is one of the biggest public health challenges.

Here's how antibiotic use in animals affects humans. If antibiotics are given to food animals, the antibiotic may kill most or all of the bacterial infection. If some bacteria survive, they become antibiotic-resistance bacteria. When animals with antibiotic-resistant bacteria are slaughtered and processed, the resistant germs can contaminate the meat. Even before slaughter, the resistant germs can make their way into the soil and water through manure.

The FDA approves antibiotic use in animals to treat sick animals, to control disease spread if some other animals are sick, and to prevent disease in animals that are at risk of becoming sick. As of 2017, drugs that are important to human health—the so-called medically important drugs—are no longer allowed to be used for growth promotion or feed efficiency in the United States.

What about the "antibiotic-free" food label? That's an interesting question, especially since there is no single definition for what this means. Moreover, the label is not approved by the United States Department of Agriculture (USDA), so there is no way to ensure that food animals do not carry antibiotic-resistant bacteria. The best we can do is follow four food safety steps to try and prevent getting sick from eating any food that might be contaminated.

Those four food safety steps to follow at home are clean, separate, cook, and chill. This means to clean your hands, food surfaces, and food. Separate refers to avoiding cross contamination by keeping raw meat, poultry, and eggs separate from other foods. Cook all foods to the right temperature to kill germs, and chill perishable food promptly. Foods should be refrigerated below 40°F and all food should be thawed in the refrigerator or in the microwave and never on the counter.

Milk

Let's turn our attention to cows and milk. For humans, cows, and other animals, milk is the first food. About 10,000 years ago, harvesting milk from other animals was discovered. If we look at cows and humans, we are both mammals. In order for both species to produce milk, hormones are necessary. Specifically, hormones of pregnancy are needed to signal to mammary glands in breasts (humans) and udders (cows) to begin milk production. Without these hormones, milk is not produced. Suckling encourages and continues hormone production and thereby milk secretion. This is called a positive feedback loop: suckling causes more milk to be produced → more milk in turn enables suckling → which causes more milk production. One event amplifies the other. Even women who have not been pregnant or given birth can stimulate milk production in the breasts. This is often done for women who adopt infants and want to breast feed.

If you've never thought about how cow milk production occurs, it might be good to know that the same positive feedback that occurs for humans is also true for cows. Cows must either be pregnant, have suckling calves, or be given hormones for milk production to occur. The common hormone used—and approved by the Food and Drug Administration (FDA)—is bovine somatotropin (bST), a growth hormone that is normally secreted by the pituitary gland. Research has shown that this hormone increases milk production, is safe for treated animals and people consuming animal products, and it does not harm the environment. The trade name for the most commonly used bST is Posilac. Note the letters "lac"—referring to lactation—in the name. In reality, how does this work? Dairy farmers can buy Posilac over the counter. About two months after the cow has a calf, the cow is injected with Posilac. Treated cows are given this synthetic hormone for about 8 months of the year after having a calf. Typically, cows lactate for about eight months. The protocol is for the milk producer to stop milking the cow after 10 months. This is followed by a two-month period of non-milking to allow the mammary gland to rest before the female cow has another calf and starts the process all over again. This is typical for milk-producing cows in the U.S. What is not typical is for mammals to drink milk after infancy or for mammals (like humans) to drink the milk of other mammals (like cows).

Tasty products like milk, butter, cheese, yogurt, and ice cream are dependent upon milk production. In fact, we know that the world loves dairy products because they are consumed by more than six billion people. And 270 million dairy cows (9.3 million in the United States alone) supply our love affair. According to World Wildlife Fund (WWF), 900 million tons of milk are produced by cows, buffalo, and other livestock worldwide for human use. India produces the most at 20 percent while the United States produces the most cow's milk at 12 percent. To understand the environmental impact, one dairy cow produces 17 gallons of manure and urine daily. See Figure 8.1, which features cows with a mountain of manure behind them, for a visual impact. This is a costly endeavor as feeding dairy herds is dependent upon water: It takes 144 gallons of water to produce one gallon of milk if you consider that 93 percent of that water is needed to grow the crops to feed the dairy cattle. Dairy cattle require a lot of food: One dairy cow eats about 100 pounds of food each day. These numbers demonstrate the significance of water and the value of properly managing wastes.

You might have heard about camel's milk as a recent addition to the mammal milk line. Camel milk has been a staple of nomadic desert people and has supported the nomadic Arab Bedouin population for millennia. The nutritional content of camel milk is similar to cow milk and varies slightly depending on species and diet. Yet, there are environmental and ethical issues of producing camel milk in the United States. Camels are not native to the United States, so they must be imported and raised under artificial circumstances, so the cost of producing camel's milk is higher than the cost of producing cow's milk.

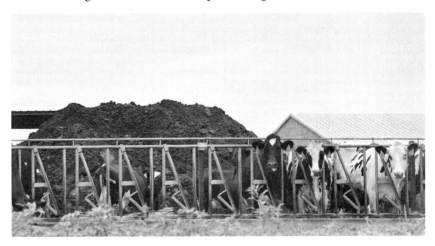

Figure 8.1 Cows feeding through a fence with a mountain of manure behind them (from Joseph Sorrentino / Shutterstock).

While on the topic of milk, what other things are important to know? Fat percentage is a good place to start. Skim milk, 1 percent milk, 2 percent milk, and whole milk all have the same amount of protein, calcium, vitamins, and minerals. Vitamin D is also added to all of them, making milk "fortified with vitamin D." What differs among them is the fat content, which in turn affects the number of calories. High-fat milks are whole and 2 percent; low-fat milks are 1 percent and skim. Fifty percent of the calories in whole milk comes from fat while 33 percent of the calories in 2 percent milk comes from fat. Skim (fat-free) milk and 1 percent milk are low fat. If you are watching fat and caloric intake, these percentages are certainly good to know.

Most milk is pasteurized, meaning that it undergoes a process that kills harmful bacteria by heating the milk to a specific temperature for a specific amount of time. In the United States, milk is pasteurized at 145°F for 30 minutes or 162°F for 15 seconds. Ultrapasteurization means the dairy product has been heated to 280°F for two seconds. Although cows eat grass in a pasture, the process has nothing to do with green grasslands, is spelled a bit differently, and is named after Louis Pasteur, who developed pasteurization. Pasteur was a French chemist and bacteriologist who discovered that high heat for a set amount of time could kill harmful organisms in milk and wine.

Most milk also undergoes homogenization. Homogenization is a process by which the fat droplets in milk are broken down (emulsified) so that they stay mixed in with the cream rather than separating. This is a physical process and no chemicals are added. In the human body, bile emulsifies fat making it is easier for enzymes to break apart molecules.

A common question that comes up whenever somebody has a cold revolves around limiting mucus (phlegm) production. Does milk cause phlegm? Phlegm is the thick, sticky substance secreted by mucous membranes of the respiratory passages. It's also known simply as mucus. When you have a cold, phlegm/mucus production increases and you get the sniffles and sticky mucus drips down the back of your throat. But milk itself does not cause your body to increase phlegm production. Irritants lining respiratory passages increase phlegm production.

Another important note regarding milk centers on its packaging. Milk in the United States is packaged in opaque plastic jugs or plastic-coated cardboard containers because light destroys riboflavin and vitamin A. If the containers were clear, the light would make the milk less nutritious. However, as little as three days in your grocer's dairy case also lessens the nutritional value as the light causes nutrient breakdown, leading to spoiling and souring. In many parts of the world, milk is sold in plastic bags, which diminishes packaging wastes. Once taken home, these "milk bladders" are placed in pitchers, the corners are snipped off, and the milk is then poured out. After use, it is placed back in the refrigerator until needed again.

Cow's Milk Alternatives

There are options for people who want alternatives to cow's milk, including plant-based (non-dairy) milks and goat's milk. Five popular plant-based milks are almond, coconut, oat, rice, and soy. Another popular milk that is neither cow nor plant-based is goat's milk. Cow's milk alternatives are good for people who have dairy allergies, are lactose intolerant, or have environmental concerns. Remember that lactose is milk sugar that requires the enzyme lactase to digest it. Some people are lactose intolerant or lactose sensitive, so they avoid lactose-based milk. But the plant-based options are also controversial because they are highly processed, and they are marketed as "milk" products, although they do not contain milk.

Breaking it down, almond milk is made from ground up almonds and water. It is a particularly good alternative for people with lactose, soy, or gluten sensitivities, plus, it has anti-inflammatory properties and antioxidant properties. Sugar and nutrients are added, but low-sugar varieties are available. Another dairy-free option is coconut milk, which is made from the flesh of coconuts. Coconut milk is rich in magnesium, iron, and potassium. A word of caution: Coconuts are indirectly related to walnuts, so people with walnut allergies could have an allergic reaction to coconut milk. Oat milk is a whitish liquid with a creamy texture made from oat grains and water. As you might expect, it tastes like drinking oatmeal. An added benefit of oat milk is that it is high in fiber. It's a relative newcomer to the non-dairy milk market as it was developed around 1990 by Swedish scientist Rickard Öste. Öste was researching sustainable food systems and lactose intolerance when he created oat milk, ultimately founding the commercial producer of oat milk, Oatly.

Rice milk is made from rice grain—mostly brown rice—and water. Soy milk is another whitish drink made by boiling ground soybeans and producing an emulsion of proteins in natural soy oil and water. Both rice milk and soy milk have varying degrees of sweetness and commercial brands have added sugars and nutrients. Soy milk contains isoflavones, which are phytoestrogens that have estrogen-like effects. Yet, soy also has anti-estrogen effects. Studies present conflicting evidence regarding soy and its estrogenic and anti-estrogenic effects on the body. Much of the conflict stems from the variation in the way soy is studied in humans. As a nutrient dense food, it does confer health benefits and current recommendations for soy consumption are to eat soy and its products in moderation.

Goat's milk has the same amount of lactose as cow's milk, but it seems to cause less digestive issues than cow's milk in people who are sensitive to cow's milk proteins. Goat's milk is being evaluated for its anti-inflammatory and anti-allergic properties.

Breast Milk

Breast milk is tailor-made for an infant and supplies the baby with nutrients that cannot be synthesized, made in a lab, or given in formula. For example, important antibodies supplied in breast milk cannot be synthesized and added to infant formula. During pregnancy, the mammary glands of the breasts start preparing for the birth of the fetus, and immediately following birth, female breasts begin secreting human breast milk. This is known as lactation, a term derived from the Latin word *lactatio* that means *suckle*. The most abundant proteins in human breast milk are casein, alpha-lactalbumin, lactoferrin, secretory immunoglobulin (SIgA), lysozyme, and serum albumin. On the other hand, cow's milk proteins are alpha-lactalbumin, beta-lactalbumin, and casein.

Returning to human breastfeeding. Breastfeeding is recommended for the first six to 12 months of life. Infant supplements are not necessary if the mother's diet is well balanced and the infant is nursing successfully. Whereas the chief protein in breast milk is alpha lactalbumin, the chief protein in cow's milk is casein, which is also the main constituent of cheese. Breast milk also offers immunological protection. For example, breast milk protects infants from antibiotic-resistant bacteria. The first milk produced by mothers is called *colostrum* or *foremilk*. Colostrum is produced for the first few days after giving birth, and it differs from the milk produced later in that it contains more proteins and antibodies. The antibodies confer immunity to the newborn. Research also shows that breastfed babies have a reduced risk of sudden infant death syndrome (SIDS), have fewer infections, and are less likely to become obese. Breast milk also encourages beneficial gut bacteria in the infant, leading to a healthier microbiome.

Breastfeeding also confers benefits to the mother. Breastfeeding decreases the risk of breast cancer and ovarian cancer. Breastfeeding also affects the pocketbook: Women can save $1,000 or more per year when they don't have to buy formula.

Agricultural Biotechnology and Genetically Modified (GMO, GM) Food

Agricultural biotechnology is the practice of using known biological processes for the purposes of producing living organisms, parts of organisms, or to improve plants or animals. This sort of biotechnology is also used to develop specific microorganisms for particular agricultural uses. It involves genetic manipulation and applies the principles of genetics, a broad field that involves the study of heredity and the variation of inherited characteristics. Two early genetic pioneers were Charles Darwin (1809–1882) and Gregor Mendel (1822–1884). Darwin was a proponent of the theory of evolution by natural selection, the biological process whereby organisms better adapted to their environment tend to survive and are thus able to produce offspring. Natural selection is slightly different from the survival of the fittest concept. Survival of the fittest is the continued existence of organisms that are best adapted to their environment while others are becoming extinct. Mendel, considered the father of genetics, systematically bred peas and showed that characteristics could be transmitted in predictable ways by genes.

However, the principles of genetics predate Mendel and Darwin. Ancient peoples—we're talking 10,000–12,000 years ago—used genetics and their understanding of heredity to domesticate and selectively breed plants and animals. Early domesticated plants we see today include barley, wheat, and peas; and domesticated animals include dogs, goats, horses, camels, and sheep. Wheat, the most widely produced and consumed grain in the world, actually originated from three grass-like species. Yes, your bowl of breakfast cereal began as a grass about 75,000 years ago. Techniques were used to enhance yield, increase size, vary color, intensify taste, and alter the ripening season. What is wrong with any of this? Several of today's greatest controversies center on cloning, genetically modified (GMO, GM) foods, and biotechnology. To many people, these terms conjure up images of Frankenstein. Let's review them and shine a light on each process.

Cloning describes the biological process in which genetically identical copies are made. It happens naturally and through genetic manipulation. Examples of natural cloning include asexual reproduction (cell division) in bacteria and sexual reproduction in humans. Bacteria produce genetically identical offspring from a copy of a single cell from the parent bacterium. This type of cloning enables bacteria to divide rapidly. To illustrate, the common bacteria that lives in our intestines, *Escherichia coli*, can divide every 20 minutes. The growth rate is exponential: If one bacterium divides every 20 minutes, within seven hours 2,097,152 bacteria will be produced! You can see why eradicating a bacterial infection can be challenging. Humans, on the other hand, reproduce through sexual reproduction so the numbers are much smaller. Human identical twins are examples of genetic clones.

Sometimes it is hard to know the origin of a particular food. For example, the produce aisle at the grocery store had a section with Autumn Glory apples from Washington grower, Domex Superfresh. The flavor profile stated that the "apple is very sweet and crisp with hints of cinnamon and subtle notes of caramel." Who wouldn't want to try that, right? It did indeed taste like it was advertised, but how did that happen? Domex Superfresh Growers are committed to sustainability and their website states that they do not grow genetically modified fruit. Instead, they created the fruit variety by cross-pollinating two or more fruit tree varieties to get the taste they wanted.

Many in the mainstream shun genetically-modified anything because people think gene manipulation is "unnatural" or "harmful" or is an attempt to breed super-humans or to create designer babies. Perhaps much of this fear or reluctance to embrace genetically-modified products is because it reminds people of the eugenics movement. Superficially, that is understandable. Yet, there is benefit to genetic modification. Nature itself modifies genes without any scientific help. Some animals and plants that exist today are not like the fauna and flora of yore because of genetic modification. Many have undergone genetic alteration to increase disease resistance, nutritional value, and yield. That said, the ethics of gene editing must always be considered.

Are you familiar with the Green Revolution? This is not the same as "going green" or the "Green New Deal," the trend toward being more environmentally conscious and legislation that supports environmental responsibility. The Green Revolution, also known as the Third Agricultural Revolution, was the application of research and genetics to increase crop production in developing countries between 1930 and

1960. Examples include high-yield crops, dwarf wheat, new methods of cultivation, fertilization and mechanization, and hybridized seeds. A key innovator in the Green Revolution was American geneticist, agronomist, and humanitarian, Norman Borlaug (1914–2009). His work in developing semi-dwarf, high-yield, disease-resistant wheat varieties improved food availability in Mexico, Pakistan, and India. For his achievements, he was awarded the Nobel Peace Prize (1970), the Presidential Medal of Freedom (1977), and the Congressional Gold Medal (2006). This is an example in which molecular genetic methods were used to secure food for swaths of people across several countries and thwart hunger. Genetically-engineered apples, corn, soybeans, and tomatoes make up our current food supply. In fact, soybeans are the number one genetically modified crop. We humans are also genetically modified through thousands of years of evolution and natural selection. For the most part, there's nothing you can do about it. You are a product of your environment.

Farmers use the tools of biotechnology to develop crops that are resistant to specific plant diseases and insects and for weed management. This is done to reduce the amount of synthetic pesticides, thereby limiting the amount in our environment. Using biotechnology can increase crop production, too. Another beneficial use of biotechnology to alter crops has been in developing plants whose purpose is phytoremediation. Phytoremediation means that the plants are able to detoxify or absorb soil pollutants to improve soil quality. The plants are then harvested and disposed of safely. Biotechnology and genetic modification aim to conserve natural resources, enable animals and people to derive more nutrients from food sources, and improve the food supply to meet demand.

A renown success story of agricultural biotechnology centers on saving the Hawaiian papaya industry. Years ago, the papaya ringspot virus threatened the population of papayas, placing the plants and the industry at risk of failing. Through biotechnology, papayas resistant to the virus were genetically engineered, saving the crop. Similar stories exist for other food crops including potatoes, squash, and tomatoes. Biotechnology has also enabled the development of crops that are richer in certain vitamins, can be grown in particular soils, or that can withstand drought. The last year for which statistics were available (2012), 88 percent of corn, 94 percent of cotton, and 93 percent of soybeans in the United States were biotechnology plantings.

Before new products are brought to the market, several

governmental agencies work together to ensure their safety. These agencies include the United State Department of Agriculture (USDA), the Environmental Protection Agency (EPA), and the Food and Drug Administration (FDA). Whenever the federal government cuts tax dollars or relaxes any regulations concerning these entities, you should be quite concerned.

Genetically modified crops can also lift South African farmers out of poverty. Because these crops can be modified to be insect-resistant, that reduces the amount of money needed for pesticides. This leads to greater yields and profits. Since 1996, the use of GM crops has added $59.5 billion to the income of global maize farmers. Between 1996 and 2018, North American GM canola farmers earned an addition $7.1 billion. Studies have shown that using GM plants that reduce the need for pesticide sprays increases income up to six-fold.

Poisons in Our Food

Organic food is produced without the use of chemical fertilizers, pesticides, herbicides, or other artificial agents. Fertilizers are natural substances or chemicals added to soil to increase its fertility. Think of fertilizers as plant food. Pesticides are substances used to kill (-*cide* means *to kill*) insects and other organisms that are harmful to plants. Herbicides are toxic to plants and are used to destroy unwanted vegetation. Think of herbicides as weed killers. But even organic foods are subject to these substances because environmental factors and vectors, like wind and other insects and animals carry chemicals from plant to plant.

Unfortunately, herbicides do make their way into our food supply. In the United States, the most widely used herbicide is Roundup, a broad-spectrum systemic herbicide that contains the chemical glyphosate. Glyphosate is particularly effective against perennial weeds and you may have spritzed some in your own garden. The chemical is found in over 750 products and has been around since 1974. And here's where it gets sticky and tricky. The huge business behind Roundup was Monsanto, who also developed genetically modified crops that could withstand spraying with Roundup. In June 2018, the German company Bayer completed its acquisition of Monsanto. So farmers had a plant that could withstand the poison, which was extremely effective at killing the weeds around the plant. This means that genetically modified crops have higher concentrations of glyphosate. Then, in 2015, the World Health Organization (WHO) determined that the active ingredient in Roundup, i.e., glyphosate, is "probably carcinogenic to humans." Fast forward to June 2020, when Bayer agreed to pay more than $10 billion to settle lawsuits over claims that Roundup caused cancer.

An analysis by the Environmental Working Group (EWG) found glyphosate in 21 cereal and snack products. According to the group's website, EWG is a non-profit, non-partisan organization dedicated to protecting human health and the environment with breakthrough research and education to drive consumer choice and civic action.

Human exposure to glyphosate has increased as more people eat GMO corn, soy, wheat, and oats. In a study of people living in the San Diego, California, area, measurable amounts of glyphosate have been found in the population. Study data are conflicting, which makes knowing how much glyphosate is safe difficult. A 2015 study by the International Agency for Research on Cancer (IARC) found that glyphosate exposure might cause cancer, but another study by the European Union found that glyphosate exposure was too low to pose a health risk.

Like microorganisms that change to thwart the effects of antibiotics, plants do the same. Thus, herbicides lose their effectiveness. Which leads us to another herbicide, dicamba. Dicamba has been on the market for a long time, but farmers are using it in place of other herbicides, which aren't working in their battle to combat damaging weeds. Unfortunately, this product is volatile and thus capable of spreading, polluting around 4 percent of U.S. soybean fields in 2017. Much of what we know about the safety of dicamba in our food supply comes from animal studies and not human studies.

Bayer is now the parent company of both Roundup and dicamba. Bayer has asked the EPA to allow the expansion of dicamba use to cover corn. This is happening despite a lawsuit brought about by over 1,000 farmers suing the company for damage to their crops as a result of dicamba drift. Bayer is a multinational company and one of the largest pharmaceutical companies in the world. Yet, in June 2020, Bayer announced it would spend up to $400 million to settle claims that dicamba can drift from its spraying site to other crops and cause damage. Add to this amount another $820 million that is being set aside for lawsuits linked to polychlorinated biphenyls (PCBs) that make their way into the water supply. In 1979, toxic PCBs were banned in the United States.

So how can we protect ourselves from consuming herbicides? The best we can do besides washing food is to buy locally from farms that engage in sustainable farming practices.

Sustainable Farming Practices

One way to protect the environment, expand the Earth's natural resources, maintain soil quality, and improve soil fertility is to use methods of sustainable agriculture. According to the National Institute of Food and Agriculture, part of the USDA, sustainable agriculture aims to increase farm income profits, promote environmental stewardship, enhance the quality of life for farm families and communities, and increase human food production and fiber needs.

Just as nutrition science is a relative newcomer in the scientific arena, agroecology is a new field of research devoted to the science of managing farms and ecosystems. Science is not static and new sciences are invented as more tools become available or they evolve as society changes. Future generations won't know a time when there wasn't such a field.

Sustainable isn't the same as organic. Although they are oftentimes close, current organic standards leave room for some practices that are not the best from a sustainable perspective, and some farmers using sustainable practices qualify for USDA certification. And some farmers using sustainable practices who could qualify for USDA organic certification may not choose to pursue it. Becoming a certified USDA organic operation is a multistep process that includes submitting an application and fees. The USDA's website provides instructions for becoming USDA organic certified. USDA organic products must meet these requirements:

1. Produced without excluded methods (genetic engineering, ionizing radiation, or sewage sludge).
2. Produced using allowed substances from the National List of Allowed and Prohibited Substances (National List).
3. Overseen by a USDA National Organic Program-authorized certifying agent, following all USDA organic regulations.

As you can see, it's a complicated, complex ordeal to have the USDA organic certification. So can products be labeled "organic" but not be certified? That's an excellent question and here's what the USDA has to say about that:

Overall, if you make a product and want to claim that it or its ingredients are organic, your final product probably needs to be certified. If you are not certified, you must not make any organic claim on the principal display panel or use the USDA organic seal anywhere on the package.* You may only, on the information panel, identify the certified organic ingredients as organic and the percentage of organic ingredients.

You can search for USDA organic certified farms and businesses using the USDA's Organic Integrity Database.

The term *sustainable* keeps coming up. What are these sustainable practices? Key practices center on diversification and keeping things simple by mirroring nature. Here are some practices used by sustainable farms:

1. Rotating crops and planting diversity. This involves multi-year crop rotation schedules and intercropping in which a mix of crops is grown in the same area.
2. Planting cover crops. This involves planting cover crops in the off-season to protect the soil, prevent erosion, replenish nutrients, and reduce herbicide use. Common cover crops include clover and hairy vetch, a species of wild pea.
3. Using no till or reduced tillage. When traditional plowing is used to prepare fields for planting, much of the soil gets lost from wind and runoff. With no-till or reduced till methods, seeds are planted directly into the soil.
4. Using integrated pest management (IPM). This involves using mechanical and biological controls to reduce or eliminate the use of chemical pesticides.
5. Integrating livestock and crops. This is a practice in which animals and crops should be integrated, versus keeping the two separated from each other.
6. Using agroforestry. This involves mixing trees and shrubs in the fields to provide shade and shelter for plants and animals. This reduces water resources.
7. Managing whole systems. This involves creating an ecosystem in the land that supports the entire landscape. Planting riparian buffers (vegetation along riverbanks) and prairie strips (grassland areas) controls soil erosion, reduces nutrient runoff, supplies habitat for pollinators, and increases biodiversity.

* Some operations are exempt from certification, including organic farmers who sell $5,000 or less.

Cattails are good plants used to prevent soil erosion because they have a dense root system. When placed between crops and open water such as rivers, lakes, and ponds, they filter toxins out of the runoff and their nitrogen-fixing bacteria in their roots absorb the nutrient and redistribute it to the surrounding soil. However, they must be closely managed as they are invasive and form dense vegetation that can impede water flow.

If you'd like to learn more about cultivating a sustainable future, check out Shelburne Farms in Shelburne, Vermont, and Polyface Farms in Swoope, Virginia. Both have strong sustainable farming missions, give tours, and educate people worldwide on best practices. We only have one planet. It behooves us to take care of it because in so doing, we also take care of ourselves.

9

The Skinny

Other Popular Diets, Fads,
Wonderments and Myths

Popular Diets

By 2030, half of the U.S. population will be obese with one in four Americans registering as "severely obese" with a body mass index over 35. For the sake of reference, this equates to about being 100 pounds overweight. Despite this statistic, many people want to lose weight and dieting tops New Year's resolutions. To discuss every fad, diet, food trend, or dietary supplement is beyond the scope of a single chapter. However, summary descriptions of some of the most popular diets are given. Market leaders include Weight Watchers (now referred to as "WW" or "myWW," or "Weightwatchers Reimagined"), Jenny Craig, and Nutrisystem. Very-low-calorie or low-calorie meal replacement programs include HMR (Health Management Resources), Medifast, and Optifast. Self-directed programs are Atkins, Biggest Loser Club, eDiets, Lose It!, and SlimFast. Each of these offers counseling, nutrition education, and portion control.

A 2020 study published in *BMJ* compared 14 popular named weight loss programs and found that each one produced some weight loss and blood pressure reduction during the first six months. However, after a year, the effects of the diets had diminished, leaving only one diet as a clear frontrunner: the Mediterranean diet. This diet significantly lowered LDL cholesterol at the one-year benchmark. None of the diets had any significant effect on HDL cholesterol or C-reactive protein, which is a marker for inflammation. Again, this underscores the point that we need to adopt a healthy eating lifestyle that we can stick with over time. Here is an accounting identifying those of key interest.

Weight Watchers, Jenny Craig and Nutrisystem

Weight Watchers, now rebranded as WW, is a company that was started in the 1960s and relies on a network of dieters who meet in person or online and support each other emotionally while also providing nutrition education. Oprah is a fan and partial owner. The company is trying to change its image from a diet company to a health and wellness company. This makes sense because its approach is sound: lose weight through healthy eating, exercise, and a network of support.

Jenny Craig is another market leader in online weight loss programs. With Jenny you get a dedicated personal consultant, delicious food, and real results—per the website. As with most weight loss programs, it's a mixed bag of success stories and attrition. You should be seeing a common thread.

Nutrisystem is an online commercial weight loss company that provides food and services. Their website states that their "proven approach combines three key features for healthy weight loss" and it "includes easy-to-prep meals delivered to your door using chef-created delicious food that is perfectly balanced to put you in fat-burning mode." Sound too good to be true? Of course it does, because it is! As with many gimmicks, the data don't support the claims. While initial results are promising, long-term results are not sustainable. This is not how we were intended to live our lives. Plus, it is quite expensive!

South Beach Diet

The South Beach diet is similar to the low-carb diet discussed in Chapter 4. It focuses on controlling insulin levels by eating unrefined slow carbohydrates. It does have merit.

Raw Food Diet

The raw food diet looks a lot like the vegetarian diet and does make a lot of sense. This diet suggests that three-fourths of a person's diet should consist of foods and beverages that are not processed, are completely plant-based, and if at all possible, organic. There are four main types: raw vegetarians, raw vegans, raw omnivores (one eats food of both plant and animal origin), and raw carnivores (one eats the flesh of animals). A cautionary note: eating raw can be dangerous because microbes inhabit raw meats and these microbes can cause illness if they are not killed through cooking.

Mediterranean Diet

The Mediterranean diet (discussed briefly in Chapters 5 and 6), focuses on plant-based food, fresh fruit, nuts, whole grains, seeds, and olive oil. Additionally, cheese, yogurt, fish, poultry, up to 4 eggs per week, and small amounts of red meat are consumed. Plus, wine. In fact, low to moderate amounts of wine are a staple. This diet has been studied extensively and does seem to improve one's quality of life by lowering the rates of various diseases.

People who follow patterns of eating that closely resemble the Mediterranean diet have better cardiovascular profiles and perform better on cognitive function tests. Older people following such a diet were also less frail. For many people, this dietary eating pattern worked as well as, or better than medications for improving heart and brain health and reducing diabetes risk.

In patients who already have type 2 diabetes, eating a Mediterranean diet lessened the development of diabetic retinopathy. The retina is a layer of nervous tissue in the back of the eyeball that is sensitive to light and triggers impulses that pass through the optic nerve to the brain, where visual images are formed. Diabetic retinopathy is an eye disease in which the retina is damaged, leading to blindness. It affects up to 80 percent of people who have had diabetes for 20 years or more. A meta-analysis of scientific studies on the health outcomes of a Mediterranean diet with no restriction on fat intake showed that people following such eating were less likely to suffer heart attacks, strokes, diabetes, breast cancer, and colorectal cancer. This diet is a winner!

Gluten-Free Diet

Gluten-free diets are quite popular today. You see gluten-free items listed on menus, on food labels, and anywhere else food is consumed or purchased. Despite this, there is much misinformation surrounding gluten. Let's begin by explaining what gluten actually is. Gluten is an insoluble protein found in wheat, barley, and rye. As an insoluble protein, it cannot be dissolved. You know gluten as the protein in flour that allows flour to rise during baking, and it is responsible for the elastic texture of bread dough. Common gluten-free grains are rice and quinoa (which is actually a seed from the plant).

In many instances, gluten causes little trouble. However, in people with celiac disease, it is quite troublesome. Celiac disease is an autoimmune disorder in which the small intestine is sensitive to gluten, causing the immune system to attack the intestinal lining. This in turn leads to difficulty digesting food, chronic inflammation of the intestines, diarrhea, malabsorption, and steatorrhea (fatty stools). Malabsorption causes nutritional deficiencies resulting from the inability to absorb nutrients, which in turn leads to weight loss, failure to thrive, short stature, and death. For people with celiac disease, gluten is totally off the menu.

Identifying celiac disease has an interesting history that dates back to the mid–1940s. Before the underlying cause was known, people could literally starve to death, even though food was available because their reaction to gluten prevented the absorption of other nutrients as well. Doctors tried experimental diets consisting of mussels, bananas, and rice. While this helped, it certainly wasn't a sustainable diet. Enter an era of famine.

The discovery of celiac disease has its roots in famine during World War II and a dedicated Dutch pediatrician, Dr. Willem-Karel Dicke. During the winter of 1944–45, people in Holland were starving. The period was known as *Hongerwinter*, the Dutch word for "hunger winter." During this horrific time, food was scarce to non-existent and what was available was nothing more than watery soup. Bread was no longer a staple. At the same time, physicians were noting that their patients with celiac disease, though famished, were no longer suffering from the malabsorption and its effects and actually could gain weight.

After the war ended and food supplies were restored, including wheat and bread, Dr. Dicke noticed the return of celiac symptoms in his patients. Over the next five years, Dr. Dicke continued experimenting with wheat-free diets and ultimately made the connection between gluten and celiac disease. These findings led to our modern-day treatment of gluten avoidance for celiac patients.

For the rest of the population, going gluten free seems to be a food trend. Moreover, sticking to a gluten-free diet is difficult. When scientists analyzed the feces and urine of people who were "gluten-free," they discovered that people were still getting anywhere from 150 mg to 400 mg of gluten per day. This is a bit alarming. Even if you are trying to be gluten-free, it may be hidden in foods, medication, and cosmetics such as lipstick.

Let's circle back to the gluten-free food trend. To be clear, people with celiac disease should absolutely avoid gluten. But lots of people have jumped on the gluten-free food train because it has been touted for weight loss, or because their favorite celebrities declared themselves gluten-free, or for whatever reason. Manufacturers have paid attention, too, and myriad gluten-free products are on store shelves. We have gluten-free bread, pasta, cereal, and other items. Marketing also plays a role as the shelves also contain products like milk advertised as being gluten-free. Of course, milk is gluten-free! It doesn't come from barley, rye, or wheat! But sometimes the gluten-free label exists because food may be produced on the same equipment that handles gluten-containing products, so there is a risk of cross contamination. Gluten-free options do make it nice for people with celiac disease and for others who are limiting carbohydrate intake.

According to a study in 2016, the number of people who actually have celiac disease had not changed significantly between 2009 and 2014: About one person in 150 has the disorder. During this same five-year time period, people following a gluten-free diet tripled! Interestingly, people on a low-gluten diet report feeling better. This may be a case of the placebo effect or because they are actually choosing more nutritious foods.

Many people opt for gluten-free as a weight loss option although going gluten-free is not a proven method to lose weight. Many gluten-free foods have added sugar and other refined carbohydrates as flavor enhancers, so they have more calories than the wheat food they are replacing. Instead, limit the amount of refined carbohydrates—like the kind in junk food.

Fasting

Fasting is abstaining from food. There are different types of fasting and all prohibit eating of some sort. For many people, fasting is also part of religious practice or ritual. With fasting come metabolic adaptations to caloric restriction. It is not bad to fast; early weight loss occurs along with decreased insulin secretion, and fluid balance may be affected.

One form of a fasting diet is called the "detox diet" or "cleanse."

Usually these involve not eating solid food for a day, then the next day eating fruits and vegetables, and then maybe taking an enema. The purported goals are to clear toxins, improve energy, and help you lose weight.

Thinking logically about the detox/cleanse, and using the basic principles of physiology, we know that the body already has systems in place for "detoxing." The liver and kidneys deal with metabolic wastes, while toxins and waste products are eliminated by the digestive and urinary systems. So fasting isn't going to clear your body of toxins. On the other hand, it's always good to have fruits and vegetables in your diet, so that part makes sense. Fasting is okay if you are already healthy to begin with, but relying on a strict diet isn't a sustainable practice for keeping off excess weight. Do you really want to spend the rest of your life having every thought centered on food? If you want a good "clean out," drink plenty of water and get at least five servings of fruits and vegetables per day while eating foods that are high in fiber. Probiotics and prebiotics are also important to add to the mix.

That said, there is some sound science that supports intermittent fasting such as only eating during a specified 8-hour window during a 24-hour cycle. This is known as the 16-hour fast and referred to as 16:8. Research is showing it to be an effective weight-loss strategy and perhaps can improve health by delaying type 2 diabetes and Alzheimer's disease while enhancing memory, adding years to your life, and treating various cancers (by starving cancer cells). Most studies have been done in animals and many done in humans have been defacto: people whose circumstances have caused starvation. Fasting also comes with rebound binging because let's face it, food is good.

Fasting diets also mirror caloric restriction (CR) diets done over the years. Some people on caloric restriction diets do lose weight, but just slightly less than those on fasting diets. It's important to keep in mind that calories are important for overall body function and we humans die when our body mass index (BMI) hovers around 12. Here's a chart outlining calorie requirements to sustain life, lose weight, or reach the danger zone.

Calories and Sustaining Life

Sex	Average Daily Calories Needed	Daily Calories to Lose Weight	Daily Calories Danger Zone	Fatal BMI
Male	2,500	1,875	1,500	13
Female	2,000	1,500	1,200	11

Blood Pressure Lowering Diets— High Dairy Diet and DASH Diet

We spent quite a bit of time talking about dairy in the previous chapter. But might a high dairy diet lower your blood pressure? The answer is, it might. In a study of overweight middle-aged adults conducted in the Netherlands, researchers found that volunteers who ate five to six servings of low fat dairy products each day lowered their systolic pressure by five points and their diastolic pressure by three points. For the purposes of the study, one serving amounted to one cup of low-fat milk or buttermilk, three-quarters of a cup of low fat yogurt, and one slice of low-fat cheese. For a refresher on blood pressure, normal blood pressure is around 120/80; 120 is the systolic pressure and 80 is the diastolic pressure. Systolic pressure is the pressure in the arteries when the heart contracts while diastolic pressure is the pressure in the arteries when the heart relaxes. The sample size of the study was small with only 52 participants, but these findings are significant.

Another diet that has withstood the test of time for lowering blood pressure is the Dietary Approaches to Stop Hypertension (DASH) diet, discussed in Chapter 5. The DASH diet is low in sodium and rich in fruits, vegetables, low-fat dairy products, fiber, calcium, potassium, and magnesium. Note that the DASH diet is also rich in dairy. DASH diets have been found to significantly reduce blood pressure in people with and without hypertension.

Grapefruit Diet

The grapefruit diet, also known as the "Hollywood diet" or "10-day diet," or "10-pounds-off diet," has been around since the 1930s. Its premise—and promise—is that you eat one grapefruit at every meal because grapefruit contains a fat-burning enzyme. This diet lasts 10–12 days with two days off, and then it starts all over again. There is no scientific evidence to support this diet.

There is scientific evidence that shows eating grapefruit or drinking grapefruit juice while taking some medications can affect the drug's metabolism. For example, statins are popular drugs used to lower cholesterol. Grapefruit can interfere with protein enzymes that metabolize statins, causing more medicine to be absorbed in the body, increasing the amount of drug in the bloodstream, and risking a possible overdose. Grapefruit can also interfere with allergy medicine like fexofenadine

(Allegra). Fexofenadine requires a protein transporter to move the drug from the bloodstream and into the body's cells. In this scenario, grapefruit blocks the transporter, decreasing the amount of medicine in the cells, thereby reducing the drug's effectiveness.

In 1999, American singer-songwriter, Weird Al Yankovic (Alfred Matthew Yankovic), parodied the grapefruit diet in his song "Grapefruit Diet" on the album *Running with Scissors*. The song used was "Zoot Suit Riot" by Cherry Poppin' Daddies. Google it—it's a fun song!

Cabbage Soup Diet

Cabbage soup. Yum. Or not. As its name suggests, you eat cabbage soup. It is touted as a short-term weight loss diet to kick start your weight loss plan. The idea of the cabbage soup diet is to eat cabbage soup two to three times per day with other assigned foods on each day of the week. For example:

Day 1—add fruit, but no bananas
Day 2—add vegetables, but no fruit
Day 3—add fruits and vegetables
Day 4—add bananas and skim milk
Day 5—add beef or baked chicken without skin and tomatoes
Day 6—add beef and vegetables
Day 7—add brown rice, unsweetened fruit juices, and vegetables

While you will likely lose weight after eating this for a week, it's not because of cabbage but rather because you are severely restricting your calories. However, it's not a sustainable route to go. Remember that when you restrict calories, your body responds by lowering your metabolic rate. When the metabolic rate is lowered, so are the number of calories burned during digestion. Lowered caloric intake results in lowered metabolism, which leads to a plateau. This is a common occurrence with low-calorie, long-term diets. This also explains why after you quit such a low-calorie diet and begin eating normally again, you will gain weight. As you've learned so far, every day should contain healthy servings of fruits, vegetables, and whole grains. Be leery of any diets with severe dietary restrictions.

Zone Diet

The Zone Diet suggests daily food intake be divided into ratios containing 30 percent protein, 40 percent carbohydrates, and 30 percent fat. Simple meal plans include breakfast, lunch, mid-afternoon snack, dinner, and pre-bedtime snack while each plate at these meals is divided into thirds of one-third protein, two-thirds carbohydrate, and a little fat. No food is off limits but processed, refined, and high-sugar foods are discouraged. It's a decent diet that encourages healthy eating.

The Freshman Fifteen and Quarantine 15

Ahh, the "Freshman Fifteen," "First Year Fatties," "Fresher Spread," or "Fresher Five." These are terms describing the weight gain that occurs during the first year of college. Depending on whether you are in the United States, New Zealand, or Australia will determine which phrase you likely encounter. The "Five" in "Fresher Five" refers to five kilograms, which is 11 pounds.

Purported causes of the weight gain during the freshman year include (1) consuming increased calories from drinking alcohol (this despite the fact that in the United States, freshman entering college generally aren't old enough to legally drink alcohol); (2) eating high-fat and high-carbohydrate meals in cafeterias; (3) the availability of high-calorie, low-nutrient fast foods; (4) stress; and (5) decreased exercise. But what if this were all a myth? A myth that ranks up there with drinking eight glasses of water per day? Actual scientific studies have shown that despite the prevalence of the common expression, it's a myth.

Researchers found that college students didn't gain any more weight during their freshman year than did those people who didn't attend college right out of high school. Research has shown that college students do gain weight steadily during their college years, just like non-college students over the same time frame. Few people gain 15 pounds and some actually lose weight. So it's not college causing the weight gain. It's adulthood.

Since the novel coronavirus entered our lives, COVID-19 also had a little more in store for us. And store we did. Enter "Quarantine 15," the new phrase in our pandemic lexicon describing our weight gain during lockdown. Much like the virus itself, we're still learning more about this health issue. Thus, it is too soon to make scientific claims. But we can point to trends and what we know about stress eating.

Facebook lights up with phrases such as "quarantine 15" and #quarantineweightgain. It seems many of us gained weight as we turned to our comfort foods and drink: candy, bread, baked goods, noodles, and alcohol. During the last two weeks in March 2020, the website Lose It! reported a 255 percent increase in people eating candy! Yet, there is widespread concern about the weight gained from over-eating, sedentary behavior (hello, Netflix), reliance on packaged food, and lack of physical activity. Stay tuned for the research and findings.

Noom and Health Apps

Searching for guidance in making healthy food choices and lifestyle changes can be a daunting task. When it comes to fad foods and fad diets, we know they typically backfire because we need to establish life-long habits that fit each of us individually—no two people are alike. Many of us use Google as our guru for guidance. Google can lead us astray or to some very helpful services. And where diet is concerned, the saying holds true: "There's an app for that."

A weight-loss app that is currently getting a lot of traction and publicity is Noom. This health app is designed by behavioral psychologists; allows you to track foods you eat by searching databases of over 150,000 foods and scanning bar codes on packaged items; logs exercise, weight, blood pressure, and blood sugar; gives one-on-one health coaching during business hours; provides helpful articles and quizzes; and generates personalized caloric breakdowns. It's like having a personal coach at the ready. All of these factors are quite good, especially since it "creates long-term results through habit and behavior change, not restrictive dieting," per Noom's website. The downside is that it costs $45 per month. That's a small price to pay for good health.

Research shows that tracking our daily food intake helps us lose weight if we are trying to do so. These food diaries are good because it is surprising to learn how much food you actually consume in a day until you write it down. Other research shows that using a food tracking app helps people lose more weight than those who were simply trying to watch their diet. For really good news, a 2016 Scientific Reports study that looked at 35,000 people found that 77 percent of Noom users reported weight loss after using the app for 9 months.

Studies have also found that sharing goals within a supportive community helps people striving for weight loss to lose weight. Many popular diets do this as do other apps. In fact, you don't have to pay for an app in order to achieve the same results. There are several free health apps—not all related to weight loss—that may help you feel better and achieve personal goals. Here is a sampling: Beach Body On Demand,

Class Pass, Glo, Grokker, My Fitness Pal, Nike Training Club, Peloton Digital, and Physique 57 On Demand. The best approach is the one that works for lifetime health.

Supplements and Herbal Remedies

Like weight loss diets, supplements and herbal remedies are big business. Supplements are substances that complete or enhance something else. Supplements can also be taken to remedy a dietary deficiency. For example, if a person is deficient in vitamin C, they can take a supplement of vitamin C and boost the level. Herbal remedies rely on medicines made from plants to treat illness or disease. Store shelves are chock full of such supplements and herbs and include St. John's Wort, saw palmetto, chondroitin sulfate, glucosamine, ginkgo biloba, and vitamin E. The herbal, St. John's Wort is used for depression and may work but also has adverse interactions with many prescribed drugs. Another herbal, saw palmetto, used for an enlarged prostate may work, but its safety is uncertain. Chondroitin sulfate used for osteoarthritis and ginkgo biloba used for improving cognitive function in dementia may work, but again, the safety is uncertain. You should see a common thread here: may work and uncertain safety. Much of this has to do with the fact that supplements are not regulated by the FDA; thus, there is no way to be certain of what's in the supplement or how much of any ingredient is in the supplement. Delaying or replacing essential medical treatments that may save your life for unknown treatments is not recommended. Moreover, many herbals interact with conventional medications that do work well. This interaction may render a perfectly effective medication ineffective.

In addition to the available, powerful, mainstream medications and treatments, patients want easing of emotional distress, comfort, relaxation, and relief of physical signs and symptoms such as pain and insomnia. Even when there is no credible evidence that something can be cured by untested alternative medicine that differs from established treatment, it may nurture hope and help improve the quality of life. One repeatedly hears the word "natural" (food and herbs) as a substitute for artificial (medications). However, "natural" does not always signify safe.

Some supplements may actually be harmful if not taken with knowledge and care. For example, high doses of vitamin E and ginkgo biloba have been shown to possess anticoagulant effects and thus, can result in bleeding in patients undergoing surgery. Soy contains plant estrogens that could, under the right circumstances, stimulate the growth of breast or endometrial cancer. Some supplements may have the ability to actually counteract conventional cancer medications. St. John's Wort (often used as a mood booster) has been shown, in some instances, to lower blood levels of a drug used to treat colorectal cancer. Even the long touted and highly recommended antioxidants that have been shown to limit adverse effects of chemotherapy and radiation sometimes even make these treatments ineffective.

Nevertheless, studies are in progress to evaluate risks and benefits of integrating herbs, vitamins, and other supplements with conventional treatments. Popular studies are based on diet, body manipulations, and mind-body techniques. One easy and cheap treatment that helps many disorders is moderate exercise. Moderate exercise eases both physical and emotional symptoms of stress, and it improves strength, mobility, and range of movement.

Ongoing research at the National Cancer Institute has shown that vitamin E may inhibit cancer-causing nitrates (found in smoked and cured foods) and prevent nitrates from producing potent carcinogenic chemicals and tumors in the body. Although vitamin E may protect against the development of certain forms of cancer (particularly among smokers), the degree of protection is still unknown.

The herbal huang lian, being studied at Memorial Sloan Kettering Cancer Center in New York, contains several main compounds and numerous minor compounds. Unlike many single herbals now being used and tested (Chinese remedies appear to be a blend of many herbs), the mixture appears to kill cancer cells in the laboratory by interfering with the cells' development. It will be interesting to see what these studies ultimately reveal.

Supplements containing folic acid (a water-soluble B complex vitamin), omega-3 fatty acids (found in fish oils), and diets rich in antioxidants such as vitamin E, vitamin A, and beta carotene, may help protect or reduce the incidence of heart disease. Studies are being undertaken to compare the supplementation in pill form versus that supplied in the diet.

Research using controlled studies has found no specific herb to reduce heart attacks or strokes, but some have been shown to lower cholesterol and triglyceride levels. One should be warned that some herbals may actually be dangerous and create risks. For example, using ginkgo biloba could result in excessive bleeding if used along with blood thinners, such as Coumadin (warfarin) or heparin. Ephedra (ma huang), an herbal stimulant, may lead to dangerously high blood pressure and heartbeat irregularity.

As an antioxidant, vitamin E is considered to be one of the best natural defenses against free-radical damage. A small study in France has demonstrated that combining vitamin E with a cholesterol-lowering drug may prevent the buildup of plaque on arterial walls and may help prevent heart attacks and strokes. These results, however, are still controversial.

Coenzyme Q10 (CoQ10 or ubiquinone) is a strong antioxidant that protects the body from free radicals and aids cellular mitochondria in transforming food into ATP, the energy on which the body runs. It has been investigated for use in angina (chest pain), high blood pressure, cardiomyopathy (enlarged heart), congestive heart failure, diabetes, gingivitis (inflamed gums), heart attack and mitral valve prolapse (faulty heart valve). Keep an eye on the latest findings as they become available.

Supplemental or complemental remedies now being tested include chondroitin, chondroitin sulfate, glucosamine, and S-adenosylmethionine (SAMe). Chondroitin sulfate is often combined with glucosamine. It may help, but more research is needed. One must be careful because it may elevate blood sugar level (not good in people with diabetes) as well as promote excessive bleeding if one is also taking a blood thinner (Coumadin or heparin).

Glucosamine may reduce osteoarthritis pain and improve flexibility, particularly in the knees and hips. One must be careful here, too, since it may interfere with insulin, causing a blood sugar rise. Avoid this supplement if you are allergic to iodine or shellfish.

S-adenosylmethionine (SAMe) has been used for many years in the treatment of liver disease, osteoarthritis (particularly with pain in the knees, hips and spine), and depression. It may cause stomach upset and nausea in high doses, and in some people, it has been shown to cause anxiety, restlessness, insomnia, and even mania.

Supplements may also interfere with the action of prescription drugs. Some may cause more drug to remain in circulation while others may limit its availability. Sometimes there is a synergistic effect, which means that when the supplement and drug are taken together, each drug has an enhanced effect. Here is an alphabetical chart showing common herbal supplements with common drugs they interfere with along with the effects.

Common Supplements with Their Noted Drug Interactions

Supplement	Interfering Drug	Effects
Black Cohosh	Lipitor (atorvastatin) Tylenol (acetaminophen)	Could lead to liver toxicity
Coenzyme Q10	Coumadin (warfarin)	Increases blood clot risk
Cranberry	Coumadin (warfarin)	Increases bleeding and bruising
Echinacea	Caffeine Other drugs metabolized by liver	With caffeine: Headache, insomnia, increases shakiness With other drugs: check with your pharmacist or doctor
Feverfew	Coumadin (warfarin), Lovenox (heparin), Plavix (clopidogrel), Xarelto (rivaroxaban)	Increases bleeding
Ginger	Coumadin (warfarin) and aspirin	Prolongs bleeding time
Ginkgo Biloba	Prilosec (omeprazole), Lescol (fluvastatin), Aricept (donepezil)	Metabolized by liver, so drug effects can be decreased or otherwise altered
Ginseng	Antihypertensive drugs (blood pressure medications) Insulin Warfarin	Decrease effectiveness
Goldenseal	Antipsychotic drugs Numerous others	Check with your pharmacist about all possible interactions
Green Tea	Coumadin (warfarin) Nadolol	Coumadin: Interferes with blood-thinning Nadolol: reduces level of drug in the blood
Kava	Buprenex (buprenorphine), Butrans (buprenorphine), Probuphine (buprenorphine), Alcohol	All: respiratory distress, coma, liver toxicity
Melatonin	Muscle relaxers, antihistamines, benzodiazepine, hypnotics, St. John's Wort, kava	Increases drowsiness, increases blood glucose, affects blood clotting
St. John's Wort	Tricyclic antidepressants, monoamine oxidase inhibitors, selective serotonin reuptake inhibitors, warfarin, dextromethorphan, birth control pills, HIV medications, and others	Interactions are numerous; check with your pharmacist for any possible drug reactions

Supplement	Interfering Drug	Effects
Saw Palmetto	Drugs used to treat benign prostatic hypertrophy (BPH), birth control pills, estrogen	Interactions are numerous; check with your pharmacist for any possible drug reactions
Valerian	Muscle relaxers, antidepressants, pain medications, anxiety medicines	Interactions are numerous; check with your pharmacist for any possible drug reactions
Yohimbe	Blood pressure medicines, cardiovascular medicines	Interactions are numerous; check with your pharmacist for any possible drug reactions

Although more evidence is needed to tease out the beneficial effects of herbal treatments for osteoarthritis, the following have been tried and are still being used by some. These treatments include boswellia, turmeric (curcumin), evening-primrose oil, ginger, guggul, horse chestnut seed extract, shark cartilage, and stinging nettle. Guggul may lower blood cholesterol levels.

Regarding ginger, in addition to its soothing effects for easing nausea, some research shows that it can reduce blood pressure and ease arthritis pain. This is good news because many over-the-counter medications people use for joint pain also increase blood pressure. Ginger lowers blood pressure by blocking calcium channels. Calcium channels are involved with muscle contraction in skeletal, smooth, and cardiac muscle. For ginger to affect blood pressure, it affects the smooth muscle in our arteries, causing relaxation (vasodilation) and on our atria (heart chambers), causing depressed rate and force of contraction. Both of these events reduce blood pressure. The effects are dose dependent, and in animal studies, ginger is as effective as the prescription medication, verapamil, which is commonly used to treat hypertension, chest pain, and cardiac arrhythmias. In addition to treating cardiovascular ailments, verapamil is also prescribed for preventing migraines. This begs the question: Does ginger then help prevent migraines?

While studies have shown ginger to have analgesic effects, the evidence about ginger's efficacy in treating migraines is scarce. In a double-blind, placebo-controlled, randomized clinical trial of ginger, results showed that adding ginger to non-steroidal anti-inflammatory drugs is effective in treating migraine attacks. Patients in this study received 400 mg of ginger extract (*Zingiber officinale*) along with 100 mg of ketoprofen (given intravenously). Earlier studies have shown that using ginger powder for treating migraine attacks is comparable to treatment with cumatriptan (Imitrex), but with fewer side effects. As with many supplements, there are not many studies, but this is likely a case in which you can use ginger, and if it works, great! Just be careful if you are currently taking a prescription drug like warfarin or Coumadin because ginger interacts with these drugs and causes prolonged bleeding time.

Another problem with taking supplements is that they are not regulated by the Food and Drug Administration (FDA), which means that there is no oversight to regulate the products' contents. Per the FDA's website (www.fda.gov), its mission is to protect the public health by ensuring the safety, efficacy, and security of human and veterinary drugs, biological products, and medical devices; and to ensure the safety of our nation's food supply, cosmetics, and products that emit radiation. That in itself is a lofty list. It also does a lot more, but they can't police every product, so many supplements on the store shelves can contain whatever the manufacturer wants them to contain. Independent testing of hundreds of bottles of herbal supplements have found that many don't contain what the label says, and fillers are commonly used. Those fillers include wheat, rice, beans, and houseplants.

If you want to be assured that your turmeric supplement really contains turmeric, or any other supplement you take actually contains what it is supposed to contain, look for "USP" on the label. USP stands for United States Pharmacopeia and is a compendium of drug information published by the United States Pharmacopeia Convention, which is a nonprofit organization. In practice, this means that if a particular dietary supplement or herbal medicine has the USP label on it, this group has deemed the ingredients to be the real deal. The standards for strength, quality, and purity have been reached. Unlike the FDA, the USP cannot enforce standards. Furthermore, manufacturers must willingly allow the USP to test products. If brands have this USP marking on the label, the general public can be assured that what's on the label is in the bottle.

Healthy diets are those that contain the essential nutrients and the right number of calories. Healthy diets are also varied so they contain a variety of foods. Note the word "foods." While you may get necessary nutrients from vitamin and mineral supplements, it is always best to get them in real food. You may be thinking, a vitamin is a vitamin, right? The quick answer is yes. The real answer is yes, but. Our bodies prefer getting the nutrients from food sources. In fact, some research has shown that multivitamin supplements actually increase our mortality risk. That's right, supplementing may actually hasten our death. Of course, this is only true if you are already receiving adequate nutrition. If you are missing a specific nutrient, supplementation is necessary. The point is that studies are finding an association—not necessarily a cause and effect—between taking vitamins and supplements and earlier death.

10

Weight a Minute

Eating Well for Life

Aging and Diet

Age should be no deterrent for having vitality and zest for living. It's good to know that pain and illness are not an inevitable part of aging. You can feel better at age 60 than you did even at age 30 simply by making healthy changes in your diet and lifestyle. Yet, aging also affects our diets. Physiological changes that normally occur as we age have an effect on appetite, nutritional needs, and the ability to enjoy and process foods. Basal metabolic rate (BMR) is one change that begins around age 30. The BMR is the rate at which the body uses energy while at rest to maintain vital functions, such as breathing and keeping warm. Over the adult life span, our body temperature lowers and there is a 20 percent decrease in the BMR. The combination of a lowered BMR plus the gradual decrease of physical activity experienced by many older adults, means that older adults need fewer calories to maintain body weight than during their younger years.

Normal aging also affects how we eat. For example, as we age, saliva production lessens and chewing effectiveness is decreased. Decreased chewing effectiveness is often associated with shrinking gums, poor oral hygiene, loss of teeth, and the use of dentures. Diminishing saliva production coupled with less effective chewing may cause a person to eliminate or decrease the amount of high fiber foods in favor of foods that are softer and easier to chew. So foods with roughage are being replaced by soft, non-plant-based foods. With age, taste and smell acuity lessens, and this encourages an increase in sugar and salt intake in order to achieve taste satisfaction. Note that in order for you to taste food, you have to be able to smell it. This explains why food is often tasteless when you have a cold or stuffed up nose. Caution needs to be exercised during the food seasoning process so that people dealing with problems associated with diabetes, cardiovascular, urinary, or digestive system diseases are not put at an additional risk.

Changes in the digestive system, such as decreased intestinal motility, can adversely affect bowel elimination, resulting in difficulty emptying the bowels causing constipation. Constipation is usually associated with hard stools. Ensuring that the diet contains sufficient fluid and fiber is the usual recommendation to avoid this problem; exercise also helps. Recognizing that increasing physical activity will also increase the need for fluid intake makes it doubly important for people to make certain that they drink sufficient quantities of fluid daily. In general, it is necessary to consume enough fluid to produce at least one liter—about 1.1 quart—of clear, pale-yellow urine daily.

For many people, mealtime serves psychological as well as nutritional needs because this is a time for socialization with family or friends. When the chance to share meals diminishes, mealtimes may stop being pleasurable experiences, may become boring, and can lead to inadequate or inappropriate food intake. Some adults experience changes in living status or abilities that are directly or indirectly related to nutrition. For instance, changes in being able to move around, inadequate transportation, or insufficient monetary resources can affect the ability to obtain food necessary for adequate nutrition.

Beverage Alcohol

Time to talk about beverage alcohol again. This was discussed previously in terms of the Mediterranean diet, but alcohol is a beverage with numerous interrelationships between humans and their evolution, environment, physiology, and social activities.

Beverage alcohol is an intoxicating drink, yet we are able to drink small amounts of it without hugging the porcelain fixture. All primates have a specific enzyme that metabolizes alcohol known as alcohol dehydrogenase 4 (ADH4). Other enzymes important to metabolizing alcohol are cytochrome P450 and catalase. Moreover, variation in genes for these enzymes influence how much alcohol is consumed, the extent of alcohol-related tissue damage, and alcohol dependence. The metabolic pathways utilizing these enzymes are quite complicated as alcohol metabolism occurs at the cellular level.

Scientists suspect that the ability to digest alcohol occurred around the same time that humans began making it themselves by turning fermented fruit and other foods into booze. The earliest known alcoholic beverage residue was found in pottery used in Jiahu, a Neolithic village in China's Yellow River Valley. This residue, dating back to 7000–6000 BCE, was a mixed fermented beverage of rice, honey, and fruit.

However, ADH4 may go back even further. Using paleogenetics, the study of the past through the examination of preserved genetic material from the remains of ancient organisms, it appears humans may have developed the enzyme earlier. What is the advantage to this enzyme? So early humans could eat rotting fruit found on the forest floor. This may explain why humans link beverage alcohol with pleasure because it was identified with food, a necessity for life.

Genetic factors also play a role in alcohol metabolism. An example of the role genetics play is seen in alcohol's differing effects among diverse populations when given equivalent amounts of beverage alcohol. Asian and Native American populations have a lower alcohol tolerance than do European populations as a result of genetic differences related to alcohol dehydrogenase production.

To understand this, we once again need to look at evolution. Scientists refer to beverage alcohol as dietary ethanol or ethyl alcohol. And they use the shorthand, CH_3CH_2OH. Beverage alcohol does not fit into our standard food categories. It is not a carbohydrate, but carbohydrates are necessary to make alcohol, which is formed by anaerobic metabolism. Anaerobic metabolism means that no oxygen is required. Alcohol is metabolized into acetic acid and aldehyde, and the average rate to remove alcohol is about seven grams/hour, which is roughly one drink per hour.

Alcohol is made by fermenting sugars that are obtained from natural sources, such as grain, grapes, and potatoes. The proof number on an alcoholic beverage represents the percent by volume of ethanol. For example, 100 proof = 50 percent ethanol by volume. In the body, small amounts of ethanol act as a mild central nervous system (CNS) stimulant. Larger amounts cause CNS depression.

As a substance, it is a toxin. We don't need it, yet we can drink it in very small amounts without getting sick. Too much, however, and we're drunk and sick. Alcohol dehydrogenase is produced in the stomach. While all primates have alcohol dehydrogenase, not all primates can metabolize alcohol equally. Paleogeneticists sequenced genes from modern day primates and analyzed how they evolved over time. Alcohol dehydrogenase was found in primates 50 million years ago. These primates could metabolize small quantities of ethanol slowly. However, about 10 million years ago, a single genetic mutation occurred within our common ancestors, chimpanzees and gorillas. The alcohol dehydrogenase proteins in these primates was much more efficient at metabolizing ethanol. This change occurred at the same time as an abrupt climate change, which also altered the ecosystem and food sources. This "advanced" protein would have enabled early primates to eat rotting, fermenting fruit and survive.

Many factors must be considered for alcohol metabolism. The liver is the main organ for metabolizing alcohol, creating first-pass metabolism. This means that the liver is the first organ to begin breaking down alcohol. Other organs, however, such as the brain, do not contain alcohol dehydrogenase. In this case, other enzymes, cytochrome P450, and catalase metabolize alcohol. These enzymes are found in little structures within cells called the endoplasmic reticulum (for cytochrome P450) and peroxisomes (for catalase). Alcohol metabolism influences blood alcohol concentration.

Approximately 25 percent of swallowed alcohol is absorbed across the stomach lining (gastric mucosa), while most of the remainder is absorbed along the first segment of the small intestine called the duodenum. The rate of absorption is dependent upon many factors including how quickly the alcohol is consumed, the amount and concentration consumed, the type and quantity of food present in the stomach, and whether or not other drugs, medicine, or underlying diseases are also present. About 90 percent of absorbed alcohol is converted to acetic acid and aldehyde, which is in turn converted to acetate, in the liver. Small amounts of alcohol are excreted unaltered by the lungs (accounting for the smelly breath) and by the kidneys.

The so-called "blood alcohol level" used by law enforcement agencies is derived from measuring the weight of ethanol per volume of blood, and that calculation is expressed as a percentage. For example, an ethanol concentration of 100 mg/dL corresponds to 0.1 percent. This value is a widely used percentage reported in legal definitions of alcoholic intoxication. One ounce of 100-proof whiskey, four ounces of wine, or 12 ounces of beer yield a blood alcohol concentration of about 0.02 percent in a 150-pound person. This is about the amount of alcohol that can be cleared from the blood in one hour. So consuming alcoholic beverages at a rate exceeding one drink per hour leads to a gradual increase in the blood alcohol concentration.

Interestingly, women achieve higher blood alcohol levels than men with equivalent amounts of alcohol. Why would this be? The primary reason is that, on average, women are smaller than men, so equivalent amounts produce higher concentrations. The other reason is that men produce more alcohol dehydrogenase than women. Therefore, more pure alcohol enters a woman's bloodstream. Or, to put it bluntly: women get drunk faster.

Measurable cognitive (thinking) impairment occurs at a blood alcohol level of about 0.05 percent, walking difficulty occurs at 0.10 percent, and slurred speech is witnessed at 0.15 percent. A blood level of 0.3–0.4 percent leads to unconsciousness, and respiratory arrest occurs around 0.5 percent.

Have you heard about the flood gate urination myth? This is a persistent myth stating that a person should hold off going to the restroom as long as possible when drinking alcohol because once you go, you'll have to go again and again. The belief is that the first urination somehow triggers subsequent trips to the toilet. This is not true. That first urination occurs because a hormone called antidiuretic hormone (ADH) is not being secreted. ADH is a hormone that *suppresses* urination. If it is *not* being secreted, then the body "knows" it's time to urinate. Think about this from a physiological perspective: if alcohol was necessary for our body's needs, then we would keep it. But alcohol is not necessary—remember, it is a toxin—so we have to get rid of it. If you've had too much alcohol to drink, ADH will be suppressed, and you will urinate. And urinate. And urinate. Your choice at this point is to either urinate on your own or wet your pants.

Having said all that, we still don't know how it is that you feel "drunk." What are those mechanisms? One minute you've got a little buzz going and the next, BAM! Two neurotransmitters seem to be involved, glutamate and gamma-aminobutyric acid (GABA), however, they are still being studied to work out the exact pathways involved. As a general rule, the more you drink the more likely you'll have a hangover, characterized by headache, fatigue, weakness, dizziness, shakiness, dehydration, nausea, vomiting, and a host of other awful signs and symptoms. Hangovers typically go away on their own within 24 hours. What we do know is that hangovers are no fun.

Scientists have recently discovered that gut microbes can make people drunk without drinking. A few years ago, a woman in upstate New York was charged with drunk driving although she hadn't had a drop to drink. She was later exonerated of the charge when she was able to prove that she had *auto-brewery syndrome* (gut fermentation), a rare condition in which yeast or bacteria in the gastrointestinal system produce ethanol. Endogenous ethanol production—the body's ability to produce ethanol naturally—occurs in very small quantities normally as part of digestion. However, when fermenting microbes produce copious amounts, extremely high levels of blood alcohol can occur. Auto-brewery syndrome is more common in people who have other existing conditions such as diabetes, obesity, and Crohn's disease, but it can also occur in other people without these disorders. Other people with auto-brewery syndrome often report eating a high-sugar, high-carbohydrate diet. Various yeasts (from the *Candida* and *Saccharomyces* families) and two strains of bacteria (*Klebsiella pneumonia* and *Enterococcus faecium*) have been identified that can ferment alcohol and produce enough ethanol to make a person intoxicated. These strains may also be involved with non-alcoholic fatty liver disease.

Nutritional and pharmacological treatment does exist for people with gut fermentation. Antifungal medications, antibiotics, diet modification, probiotics, and a low-carbohydrate diet are known to help. Diets that eliminate simple and complex sugars will decrease alcohol fermentation. Probiotic supplements have also been used, but their efficacy has yet to be studied scientifically.

While gut fermenting isn't that pleasant, can drinking alcohol provide health benefits? The short answer is maybe. We know surprisingly little about the health benefits of moderate alcohol use. We know a lot about health risks. It's difficult to study alcohol and its effects on people because so much research relies on patient recall and personal habits that may or may not influence any perceived benefits of drinking alcohol.

Moderate alcohol consumption is considered fairly safe. Moderate alcohol intake for healthy adults is up to one drink per day for women and up to two drinks per day for men. Beer, wine, and distilled spirits are usually the beverages considered. But how much? As a general rule, one drink is broken down as follows:

> beer = 12 fluid ounces
> wine = 5 fluid ounces
> distilled spirits (80 proof) = 1.5 fluid ounces

You are probably scratching your head reading this because there is no standardization regarding alcohol content among the beverages. Some beer might be 3.2 percent alcohol, 10 percent, more, or anywhere in between. Some studies show that moderate drinking can have cardiovascular benefits, but we know healthy diets and exercise do confer health benefits. Heavy alcohol use and alcohol abuse are linked to malnutrition; vitamin B1 (thiamine) deficiency; Wernicke encephalopathy (neurological disorder); Korsakoff psychosis (serious mental illness); liver disease and cirrhosis (liver scarring); gastritis; pancreatitis; stroke (brain attack); high blood pressure (hypertension); cancers of the mouth, pharynx, esophagus, liver, and breast; fetal alcohol syndrome for infants born to mothers who drink too much; and suicide—to name a few.

There is one potent ingredient in red wine that is receiving lots of attention and research time. That ingredient is *resveratrol*, a polyphenol with antioxidant properties and possible anticarcinogenic effects. Resveratrol is also found in peanuts and the skins of grapes, blueberries, raspberries, and mulberries. Resveratrol is also made from the phenylalanine pathway through a series of enzymatic reactions. Recall that phenylalanine is an amino acid. Drug formulations of the compound have been used for a range of conditions including arthritis, urinary tract infections, and skin inflammation. It appears to be cardioprotective, neuroprotective, and an anti-inflammatory while also affecting disease initiation and progression. In vitro (test tube) and in vivo (living organism) evidence shows that resveratrol shows promise, but more clinical trials are needed to confirm or refute its potential.

Have you ever wondered if people who live in colder, darker climates drink more alcohol than others? There aren't many published papers on the topic. Researchers collected data from 193 sovereign countries, 50 states, and 3,144 counties in the United States and found that as mean average temperature and average annual sunshine hours went down, alcohol consumption went up. Unfortunately, along with this increased drinking came more alcoholic cirrhosis. Alcohol is a vasodilator, so it increases warm blood flow from the body's core to the extremities, causing a generalized flushing and a feeling of being warm. Whether this plays a role in increased alcohol consumptions is not known. If knowing that colder climates plays a role in alcohol consumption, public health efforts could be steered toward alcohol education and other health services.

Milk Thistle

Milk thistle, also known as *Silybum marianum*, is a plant with a single purple flower and glossy marbled leaves. Its active ingredient, silymarin, is known to have antioxidant, antiviral, and anti-inflammatory properties, so it is used in herbal medicine. It is supposed to treat liver disease, prevent and treat cancer, and protect the liver from alcohol and cancer treatments. To date, its efficacy is not known, and more research is needed to conclude whether it does any of these things.

Aspirin

Aspirin is a wonder drug. We wonder about all its uses and mechanisms of action. Were it to have been discovered today, it's unlikely that it would be an over-the-counter drug. Aspirin is used to treat pain, inflammation, and fever. If given shortly after a heart attack, death risk decreases. Long-term use helps prevent future heart attacks in people who have had a heart attack, and it is used to prevent strokes and blood clots in people at high risk for such events. Tomes have been written about aspirin. It is the most widely used and among the safest medications.

The aspirin we know today dates back to the late 1890s and is associated with another common, household name, Bayer. Felix Hoffmann, a chemist at Bayer in Germany, first used aspirin to treat his father's rheumatism, a disorder marked by joint and muscle inflammation. The history of aspirin is fascinating and really predates Hoffmann and Bayer. Aspirin's key ingredient, acetylsalicylic acid (ASA), can be found in spirea, jasmine, beans, peas, clover, some grasses, and certain trees. Ancient Egyptians extracted the compound from willow bark, and Hippocrates (460–377 BCE) wrote that willow leaves and bark relieved pain and fever. Noting that aspirin helped his father, Hoffmann thought he was on to something, and Bayer began distributing the white powder to physicians to give to their patients in 1899. In 1915, aspirin was sold as an over-the-counter medication.

Today, many people take 81 mg of aspirin daily for prophylactic measures to prevent deep venous thrombosis (blood clots in deep veins), thromboembolism (moving blood clot), and generalized inflammation reduction among other things. This same dosage is typically found in baby aspirin. Have you ever been curious about the dosage level? Why 81? Why not 80? The answer harkens back to a time when the apothecary system of weights and measures was used. Apothecaries were the forerunners of today's pharmacies and the apothecary system was a system of weights based on the weight of a grain of barleycorn and abbreviated gr. It had been used for centuries in weighing medicines, but the system has been superseded by the metric system, which is based on grams. Some drugs that have been available for long periods of time, like aspirin, are rooted in this history. Standard dosing was five gr, which is the equivalent to 325 mg. Low-dose aspirin was one quarter of 325, which is 1.25 grains, which is converted to 81 mg.

Aspirin has been called the "wonder drug" because it seems to help so many ailments, and more and more benefits of taking the drug continue to be discovered. Its mechanism of action is to block the production of prostaglandins, by inhibiting COX-1 and COX-2. COX stands for cyclooxygenase, which is an enzyme necessary for prostaglandin synthesis. Prostaglandins are tissue hormones involved in blood clot formation, pain, fever, and inflammation. At least we *think* that's what aspirin does.

Aspirin also blocks thromboxane synthesis. Thromboxanes are biochemically related to prostaglandins and formed from them by COX. Thromboxanes play a role in blood clotting. If you take one baby aspirin every day for 10 days, your platelets—the cellular fragments that play a role in blood clotting—will not contain thromboxane. Your blood will still clot because it has other clotting factors, but it will take longer because without thromboxane the platelets will not clump as easily and will require a little more time. For this reason, if you are about to undergo surgery, you'll be asked to stop taking aspirin for at least 10 days prior to surgery. Other anti-inflammatory drugs such as ibuprofen (Motrin or Advil) and naproxen (Aleve) inhibit thromboxane production, too, but the effect lasts only a few hours. Acetaminophen (Tylenol) has no effect on thromboxane. New research on aspirin also suggests that aspirin's role in cardiovascular health is much broader because it has effects on thromboxane, platelets, and inflammation through pathways that may not be fully understood.

Studies are currently showing that low-dose aspirin increases survival in patients with cancer who are undergoing treatment. Other studies show that pregnant women at risk of pre-eclampsia were less likely to develop the condition when given low-dose aspirin. With so many health benefits, aspirin might be a wonder drug. However, it should not be taken without the advice of real healthcare providers.

Exercise

An ounce of prevention is worth a pound of cure. Benjamin Franklin's axiom seems as relevant today as it was in 1736 when he was advising fire-threatened Philadelphians. The prevention in our modern-day scenario refers to exercise as medicine. As sitting becomes the new smoking, it is incumbent upon us to do something. Following our six million years of a hunter-gatherer existence, we spend our days sedentary. There are no pros to this lifestyle.

Physical activity has been shown to play a role in preventing cancer of many types, including breast, colon, endometrial, kidney, bladder, esophageal, and stomach. Decreasing sedentary time (as opposed to activity itself) is associated with lowering the risk of endometrial, colon, and lung cancers. And sticking with the cancer theme, physical activity after cancer diagnosis increases survival time for patients. Of course, it's much easier to say these words then to act upon them. Likewise, it's easier for healthy people to engage in physical activity. However, physical exercise is beneficial pre-diagnosis and post-diagnosis. The American College of Sports Medicine has updated its exercise guidelines and is attempting to create an environment whereby people are as active as possible, regardless of their current health status.

In addition to cancer prevention and prolonged life expectancy post cancer diagnosis, exercise is a drug-free approach to many ailments. In many cases, exercise works *better* than medication or it *enhances* medication effects. Exercise lowers blood pressure, helps regulate blood glucose levels, improves cholesterol, and decreases stress. How does it *actually* work? That is, what are the molecular mechanisms linking exercise with health benefits?

Relative to cancer, exercise controls cancer progression through tumor-intrinsic factors. Tumors favor aerobic metabolism; with exercise they are deprived of some oxygen, thereby preventing aerobic metabolism. Simply put, exercise reduces the rate of tumor growth by starving them of necessary oxygen—you're panting too much to give up that precious oxygen to cancer cells.

Regarding blood pressure, with exercise the heart becomes stronger and thus can pump blood with less effort. This lowers the force on the arteries and in turn this lowers blood pressure.

With respect to blood glucose, glucose levels peak within 90 minutes after eating a meal. The word that is used to indicate "after eating" is *postprandial* and is derived from the word parts *post* meaning *after* and the Latin term *prandium* meaning *meal*. Exercise lowers blood glucose levels because your muscles need energy in the form of glucose to feed them. So glucose is taken out of circulation and placed in muscle cells. Regular exercise also helps the body use insulin, the hormone that transports glucose into the cell, more efficiently.

How exercise improves cholesterol is still a little uncertain. However, scientists think that several mechanisms are involved. It appears that exercise stimulates enzymes that target LDL cholesterol, thereby removing it from the blood and passing it through the liver. The liver converts the cholesterol to bile, which is excreted, and the LDL cholesterol is lowered. Exercise may also increase the protein particle size, making it harder for them to nestle in blood vessels. The optimum amount of exercise is still up for debate.

Exercise improves physical fitness, enabling the body to better able fight disease. But it also has beneficial effects on the mind. Regular exercise decreases overall tension, elevates and stabilizes mood, improves sleep, and improves self-esteem. These benefits are seen with as little as 5 minutes of aerobic exercise each day. Physical activity stimulates the production of endorphins, those feel good chemicals that are also natural painkillers. The term *endorphin* is a blend of the words *endogenous* (coming from within) and *morphine* (an analgesic). Endorphins are secreted in the brain and have a number of physiological functions, including activating the opiate receptors causing an analgesic (pain killing) effect. Five-minute workouts help, especially if you do several throughout the day. Splitting up the exercise bursts can also have some effect on appetite control.

We've all heard it: Gotta get my steps in. I need 10,000! The truth is, we should not worry about counting our steps; rather, we should just get a good walk in daily. Walking is one of the best exercises we can do to reduce disease risk and live longer. Walking is free, requires no special equipment other than comfortable shoes, and can be done throughout our lives. But where did that 10,000 step mantra come from? It actually comes from a Japanese advertisement campaign promoting a pedometer. Ten thousand steps equates roughly to five miles. Do you need this amount? Like our diets, it is not a one-size fits all tally.

Many studies have been done since 1960 to identify the walking sweet spot. The current recommendation by the CDC—and corroborated by a large Harvard study—is 7,500 steps daily. Picking up the pace to increase heart rate and breathing is also good because faster walking speed is associated with living longer. A fast pace is about three to five mph or 100 steps per minute. Recent research showed that people who walked about three miles per hour (20-minute mile) lived 15–20 years longer than those who walked two miles per hour

(30-minute mile). Besides the physical benefits, walking also positively affects brain function and can slow or decrease age-associated cognitive decline.

As we've seen throughout these pages, diet plays a bigger role in weight maintenance than does exercise. Walking does little for weight management, but avid walkers have smaller waist circumferences. This is good news because where we carry our fat impacts our health.

Very recent research also purports great news related to running and health. In a systematic review and meta-analysis with a pooled sample of 232,149 people, running is associated with a lower risk of all-cause, cardiovascular, and cancer mortality. Any amount of running just once a week was associated with 27 percent lower risk of all-cause death, 30 percent lowered risk for cardiovascular death, and 23 percent lower risk of death from cancer. There were no significant dose-response trends for weekly frequency, weekly duration, pace, and total volume of training. Higher doses of running may not be any more beneficial than just getting out there and running.

Other studies on the benefits of running have shown that 250 minutes or more of running per week could have negative effects on mortality. The Copenhagen City Heart Study followed 1,098 healthy joggers and 3,950 healthy non-joggers prospectively for two years. Their findings concluded that light and moderate joggers had a lower mortality than sedentary non-joggers, and strenuous joggers had a mortality rate that was not statistically different from the non-jogger group. Taken in total, research seems consistent in showing that people who are physically active have at least a 30 percent lower risk of death than do sedentary people. The moral of the stories: Get up and move!

Mustard for Cramps

Okay, you're inspired to exercise and all is going swell. Then, you get a killer cramp. What do you do? Without an athletic trainer on the sideline, you're often left to tough it out. Besides being an awfully painful condition in which a muscle tenses up, what exactly is a muscle cramp? From a physiological perspective, a cramp—oftentimes called a charley horse—is a strong, involuntary contraction of one or more skeletal muscles that can last from a few seconds to several minutes. In order for a muscle to contract, neurons fire and send electrical signals to the muscle causing contractions. However, we don't want our muscles "over-firing" or having sustained contractions that we can't control.

Causes of muscle cramps are varied and include exercising strenuously, being dehydrated, lack of muscle use, low calcium or potassium levels in the blood, and some medications. Some people experience nighttime muscle cramps in their legs while sleeping. Time and gentle stretching can generally relieve the pain.

Home remedies like eating a teaspoon of mustard, drinking a shot glass of pickle juice, or drinking tonic water with quinine have been touted as working well for relieving muscle cramps. But do they work? They just might. Stimulating sensory neurons in the mouth, throat, and stomach with strong flavors can interrupt muscle contractions by affecting certain neuron receptors. It's important to keep in mind that just because science hasn't figured out why something works, if it works for you and does no harm, by all means, go ahead and use it!

Pomegranates

Pomegranates are fruits with a tough, reddish outer skin and a gelatinous flesh with clusters of juicy seeds. Pomegranate flesh is a rich source of vitamin C, vitamin K, and folate. The seeds are a good source of fiber. The fruit has a rich history as well, as it is believed to have been a fruit in the Garden of Eden, it is mentioned in other religious texts, and plays a role in Greek mythology.

A commonly used non-alcoholic syrup used in mixed drinks is grenadine. Authentic grenadine is made from the juice of pomegranates with added sugar and water. Getting juice from a pomegranate is a difficult task, so modern-day grenadine is simply corn syrup with red food coloring.

There are many health claims centered around pomegranate juice, and in 2010, the FDA issued a warning letter to POM Wonderful, a manufacturer of pomegranate juice, because they made illegal claims of unproven health benefits. Since the FDA letter, more research has been done on the health benefits of pomegranate juice.

A metabolite of pomegranates called urolithin A (UA) appears to increase mitochondrial biogenesis. Urolithin A is produced by microflora in the gut during intestinal metabolism of pomegranates. Said simply, our microbiome manufactures UA when they digest pomegranates. Mitochondria are the powerhouses of our cells that manufacture ATP, the energy our body uses. This urolithin has been shown to increase the formation of mitochondria just as exercise does. Mitochondrial breakdown is a normal part of aging, and UA seems to generate more. When we exercise, the number of mitochondria in our muscles increases, and we're able to generate more ATP more effectively. Research has shown that oral consumption of UA improved mitochondrial and cellular health.

Pomegranate juice, which is rich in polyphenols, may also play a role in lowering blood pressure. It lowers systolic blood pressure by inhibiting serum angiotensin converting enzyme (ACE). Common blood pressure medications, known as ACE inhibitors, work the same way. A systematic review and meta-analysis of randomized controlled trials on the effects of pomegranate juice on blood pressure suggests that it may be prudent to include it in one's diet if you are trying to naturally decrease your blood pressure.

Eggplant

Pomegranates aren't the only healthy food found to lower blood pressure. Research confirms that eggplants, those purple egg-shaped fruits eaten as vegetables, can also lower blood pressure. Eggplant is a rich source of the neurotransmitter, acetylcholine, which affects blood pressure; thus, it is a novel functional antihypertensive food. The effects of eggplant powder on rats with hypertension showed that eating eggplant lowered their blood pressure by suppressing sympathetic (fight-or-flight) nervous activity. Subsequent studies on humans who were given eggplant powder (1.2 g/day) confirmed its blood pressure lowering power. Additionally, daily ingestion of eggplant powder not only improved blood pressure, it also improved psychological state in stressed individuals. The reason capsulized eggplant powder was used in the study was to ensure that participants were not able to tell the difference between actual eggplant and a placebo so that true randomized placebo-controlled findings were reported.

CBD

Cannabidiol (CBD) is a phytocannabinoid, a class of diverse chemical compounds found in the plant *Cannabis savita*. We know the plant as weed, cannabis, or marijuana. CBD acts on cannabinoid receptors in the body that alter neurotransmitter release in the brain. Although CBD was discovered decades ago, scientific study and clinical evidence studies using the substance are in their infancy. To be clear, CBD is not THC, the abbreviation for the psychoactive substance tetrahydrocannabinol.

It appears that CBD has no psychoactive properties, but both are extracted from *Cannabis*.

Because there hasn't been much research on THC and CBD, it has been difficult for governments to establish policies or regulations concerning its use—whether the use is medical or recreational. We do know that cannabis can have medicinal, psychotropic, and mind-altering effects. What is not known is whether CBD attenuates or exacerbates THC's behavioral and cognitive effects—or, what else it does and doesn't do.

According to the U.S. Food and Drug Administration, they are committed to sound, science-based policy on CBD. Furthermore, "It is currently illegal to market CBD by adding it to a food or labeling it as a dietary supplement."

Sleep and Sleep Aids

Like eating well, getting plenty of exercise, and engaging in life, sleep is a key component to health. We've all experienced sluggishness during the day followed by a sleepless or restless night. Yet, do you know *why* it is that we sleep? Understanding sleep has been at the crux of research for decades. What we do know is limited, but what we can't deny is the feeling of being refreshed after a good night's slumber.

Sleep is restorative and rejuvenating. What is known is that throughout the day, our cells are active. A byproduct of cellular activity is the chemical adenosine. Adenosine is part of adenosine triphosphate, ATP, the body's fuel. The basic reason we eat is to enable our cells to produce ATP. As adenosine builds up in the brain, we begin to feel tired. Caffeine blocks adenosine's action in the brain, thus it works to keep us alert. Adenosine accumulates while we are awake, but when we sleep, it is cleared from the brain. We sleep, wake up, feel alert, and start all over again.

Other physiological events also occur during sleep. While we sleep, mitotic rate increases, which means that our cells have a chance to regenerate and repair. Studies have shown that sleep, not rest, does this, underscoring the significance of actual sleep. Growth hormone release also occurs primarily during sleep. Growth hormone is secreted by the pituitary gland in the brain and its job is to stimulate growth in our cells.

Sleep also plays a role in immune function. Animals deprived of sleep lose their immune function and die within a matter of weeks.

You likely have experienced a form of immune system loss due to sleep deprivation. Here's a classic example. You've been burning the candle at both ends, feeling a little run down because you can't get everything on your to-do list accomplished. Then, bam! You come down with a cold and are down and out for a few days. This is likely nature's way of forcing a slow down for a rejuvenation. A similar scenario occurs in college students following final exams and the beginning of a break from school. It's referred to as the *let-down effect*. During stressful periods, the stress hormone, cortisol, is increased. The increased level of cortisol keeps us on high alert for any dangerous situation. The inflammatory response also ramps up. Other chemicals in our body increase because it's part of the fight-or-flight response. We're genetically programmed for this to keep us safe. When the stress goes away or diminishes, our bodies return to a normal state, cortisol levels drop, and the immune system goes back to its original state. This surge-and-fall sets the stage for illness. Of course, the solution is to avoid stress. However, in the real world, that's not possible. This is where making sure you get plenty of exercise, eating well, and practicing deep breathing can help. Deep breathing sends a signal to your nervous system to calm down; this in turn lessens stress.

Other reasons to sleep involve the architecture of our brains. Although not completely understood, sleep plays a critical role in brain development when we are young. This is likely why infants sleep 13–14 hours per day. Sleep deprivation in adults has an impact on our ability to learn and perform a variety of tasks.

Can a person train for sleep deprivation? The answer is yes. As part of their rigorous training, U.S. Navy SEALs undergo sleep deprivation training. SEALs are trained to stay awake for five continuous days. The key is to be in constant motion. With sleep loss also comes hallucinations. Studies also show that sleep deprivation performance is similar to being under the influence of alcohol.

How do we ensure that we get enough sleep? Suggestions abound. But insomnia is a very real issue that affects many people. Insomnia, derived from the Latin word *insomnis* meaning *sleepless*, is the inability to sleep. The sleeplessness can range from having trouble falling asleep to having trouble staying asleep. People suffering from the condition feel sluggish, sleepy, irritable, and depressed due to the lack of sleep. It can be acute (short term) or chronic (long term). Nonetheless, it can be quite annoying.

Numerous conditions like psychological stress, pain, menopause, anxiety, and heartburn among others can cause insomnia. Certain medications, caffeine, nicotine, and alcohol can also contribute to sleepless nights. Regardless of the cause, people turn to over-the-counter sleep aids to alleviate the problem. They are not a magical cure, tolerance can develop quickly, and many leave people tired and groggy the next day, despite having slept. Since they are commonly used, we should take a look at some popular options.

A common ingredient in some over-the-counter sleep aids is diphenhydramine. Diphenhydramine is an antihistamine (Benadryl is a common one) that is used to treat allergies, symptoms of the common cold, dizziness, and nausea. Its common side effect is sedating drowsiness. For this reason, it is used as a sleep aid and is found in Advil PM, Aleve PM, Tylenol PM, and stand-alone medications. The PM indicates that is should be taken at night. Moreover, Advil, Aleve and Tylenol contain their other pain-relieving ingredients as well: ibuprofen, naproxen sodium, and acetaminophen respectively.

Diphenhydramine is not recommended for people aged 60 and above or for children under age six. Diphenhydramine is an anticholinergic, which means it blocks the action of the neurotransmitter acetylcholine in the nervous system. Acetylcholine plays a role in memory and learning in the brain; elsewhere in the body it is necessary for skeletal muscle contractions. Long-term use of anticholinergic medications, such as those found in sleep medications, is associated with increased dementia risk.

Another antihistamine with sedative effects is doxylamine. It is a common ingredient in cough medicines and is prescribed with vitamin B6 (pyridoxine) to pregnant women to treat morning sickness. The sleep aid containing doxylamine is Unisom Sleep Tabs. It too should be avoided in people over age 60. Both diphenhydramine and doxylamine are sedating antihistamines, but diphenhydramine tends to be milder than doxylamine, which is more effective long term.

Drugs that can be potentially inappropriate for use in older adults are placed on *Beers List*. *Beers List* was formulated by geriatrician Mark H. Beers as a guideline for healthcare professionals to help improve safety of prescribing medications to older adults. The criteria were first published in 1991 and have been updated regularly through January 2019 (to date). Diphenhydramine is on the list.

A sleep aid that is not an antihistamine but rather a hormone is melatonin. The pineal gland, a tiny structure deep in our brain, secretes this hormone to regulate the sleep-wake cycle, also called the circadian rhythm. Melatonin production is regulated by natural or artificial light. If we didn't live in an industrialized world, natural sunlight would set the pattern and determine when we are awake and when we should sleep. It also sets our feeding pattern, other hormone regulation (like the previously discussed growth hormone), and cell regeneration. Food sources of melatonin, albeit very small amounts, include fruits, nuts, olive oil, and wine.

How does this regulation occur? Sunlight (or other light) is detected by the retina in our eyes, sending a signal to the pineal gland that regulates melatonin secretion. If there's plenty of sunlight, melatonin secretion is diminished; and lack of sunlight causes melatonin secretion to ramp up. Our blood level of melatonin is low during the day and high at night. Melatonin also plays a role in regulating our body temperature. Thus, at night, we get tired and our body temperature drops a little as we physiologically prepare for sleep. In the morning, sunlight is sensed, our bodies warm up a little, and we wake up. Artificial light suppresses melatonin production and disrupts this natural rhythm. For this reason, it's best to shut down devices a few hours before sleeping. Melatonin is sold as a supplement to treat insomnia or jet lag, but its efficacy as a sleep aid is unclear as scientific reports are mixed. An over-the-counter medication with melatonin is ZzzQuil.

Melatonin has also been used in patients with cancer. While studies show that it does not treat cancer, it may improve sleep quality in cancer patients. Animal studies suggest the antioxidant properties of melatonin stimulates the immune system, but it is not known if this also occurs in humans. Some human studies show anticancer, antiproliferative, and protective effects. For example, if melatonin is used along with specific chemotherapy drugs, patient survival time increased. Melatonin showed antiproliferative (decreased cancer cell numbers) effects on breast cancer cells, and it protected the heart from doxorubicin-induced toxicity. Doxorubicin (trade names include Adriamycin, Caelyx, and Myocet) is a common chemotherapy medication used to treat many types of cancer, with heart damage as one of its serious side effects.

Can fragrances help you sleep better? They just might. I say might, because using the extracts and essentials oils of aromatic plants to treat disorders and improve psychological wellbeing is known as aromatherapy. And much of what we know about aromatherapy is that it is based in pseudoscience. Obtaining evidence is difficult because designing studies that revolve around smelling something is difficult to do. Common fragrances used in aromatherapy are lavender, chamomile, and peppermint. A recent study showed that using essential oils with hospitalized cancer patients helped them sleep better. Another study showed that lavender oil could ease anxiety. A few animal studies in mice confirm that lavender oil, specifically linalool found in lavender oil, had anti-anxiety properties. Human studies on lavender oil's anti-anxiety effects show the fragrance may help to lessen the anxiety of women who are about to undergo surgery. Another study showed that lavender extract worked better than placebo in easing anxiety.

While the studies are limited, we should view aromatherapy with a bit of skepticism and with an open mind. Nice smells are relaxing. Think about chocolate chip cookies fresh out of the oven or the scent of Thanksgiving dinner cooking. Smells are strong triggers for memories, and if either of these aforementioned events gave you the warm fuzzies, chances are your anxiety level dropped a bit, too.

A relatively newcomer to the stress-relieving scene is ashwagandha (*Withania somnifera*) extract. Ashwagandha is an herb used to reduce stress and anxiety and enhance overall wellbeing. While more research is needed, the herb has shown stress-relieving effects. It appears that it acts on the hypothalamus-pituitary-adrenal axis, which is the brain to cortisol pathway. We know cortisol is a stress hormone, and ashwagandha seems to moderate stress and anxiety. Although more scientific research is necessary, early studies show no adverse reactions. PureZzzs, an over-the-counter product from the makers of ZzzQuil, contains both melatonin and ashwagandha.

Valerian is a drug obtained from the root of the common valerian plant used as a sedative. Its efficacy has been mixed, but it doesn't seem to cause side effects, which is good. What about that soothing cup of chamomile tea? Is chamomile a good sleep-inducing agent? Again, the science isn't proving it to be beneficial for helping with sleep. While anecdotal evidence suggests otherwise, scientific data don't support it. In fact, a Japanese study compared drinking hot water with drinking chamomile tea and found that relaxation scores on a self-reported survey increased after drinking either beverage. This actually makes sense because the actual ritual of preparing the tea from boiling the water, to steeping the tea bag, to wrapping our hands around a warm mug actually calms us. So, if you like doing it, and it helps you sleep, keep on sipping.

Ginger is a spicy hot, fragrant spice made from the rhizome (ginger root) of a flowering plant, *Zingiber officinale*. It has been widely used in cooking and in herbal medicine. Some herbal medicinal uses for ginger include alleviating nausea and vomiting by acting on the gastrointestinal tract. Others include as a sleep aid. On the efficacy of ginger for nausea and vomiting, ginger appears to work better than placebo. It also may be a useful alternative to antiemetic medication to alleviate postoperative nausea and vomiting. In terms of a treatment for insomnia, the research hasn't been scientifically validated yet. Many people use hot ginger tea to relax before bedtime. If the ritual works, there is no harm.

Drinking a cup of warm milk won't help you fall asleep either. The theory behind this deals with tryptophan, an essential amino acid found in milk. Tryptophan is a biological precursor to serotonin, a feel-good chemical. Serotonin levels rise when we are happy, and some drugs used to treat depression work by maintaining serotonin levels in our bloodstream. In order for tryptophan to get into our brains and convert to serotonin, it must get through the blood brain barrier, which prevents the passage of some substances and allows the passage of others. Tryptophan in foods isn't the same as pure tryptophan, because other amino acids are also present in foods that are also competing for entry into our brains. Therefore, the hypnotic effects of warm milk tryptophan don't seem to exist. This may again be a case of calming ritual, like the chamomile tea example.

These are some pharmacological and dietary methods to overcome insomnia, but shouldn't there be a simpler, natural method to ensure a good night's rest? Perhaps a sleep routine would be helpful? It turns out that a purported habit known as *sleep hygiene* has been around since the 1970s. Sleep hygiene involves behavioral modifications and environmental practices to help overcome insomnia. The regimen involves establishing a regular sleep schedule; limiting stress; exercising, but not within two hours of bedtime; avoiding alcohol, caffeine, and other stimulants within a few hours of bedtime; shutting down the computer and work-related activities close to bedtime; using the bed for nothing but sleep and sex; limiting naps; and having a dark, peaceful sleep space. These all seem like good things; however, the actual science behind it is limited and not conclusive. Individual sleep hygiene programs do seem effective, but direct effects on the general population are not known. Sleep hygiene has also been studied in elite athletes. Findings here conclude that "based on associations between sleep hygiene, sleep quantity and sleep quality, it is suggested that improvement in critical sleep hygiene practices, such as regular sleep-wake patterns and reducing psychological strain, may help to further optimize sleep."

Should sleep really involve a pharmacological remedy? Do we need to medicate sleep? One proven non-medical sleep intervention is exercise. In addition to other health benefits of exercise, a good body workout helps you fall asleep quicker and improves sleep quality. Scientists aren't sure of the mechanism linking exercise with sleep, but it may be related to endorphin release. As little as 30 minutes of moderate aerobic exercise may be all it takes. Digging deeper into all the research, we're learning that some of us are just better sleepers than others, and if you find a regimen that works, then stick with it!

Balanced Diet

As we have learned, nutrition is the supply of nutrients that our cells need to keep us functioning. We have macronutrients, which we need in large quantities, and micronutrients, which we need is small quantities. Energy comes from the macronutrient class: carbohydrates = four calories per gram, proteins = four calories per gram, and fats = nine calories per gram. Other important macronutrients are fiber and water; vitamins and minerals provide no energy but make up our micronutrients. All are important!

Overall, we need balance. Foods and fluids provide the essential nutrients and energy calories that enable efficient body functioning. Fluids, with or without nutrients, play a vital role in regulating body temperature, elimination, and circulation. For most adults, 2.1 quarts of fluid per day is sufficient for effective body functioning. Fluid can come from beverages or from the water found in solid food. We must choose foods that are high in nutritive value to obtain adequate nutrients and maintain one's proper weight. Moreover, the margin of error, or the proportion of the diet composed of empty calories that you can afford to consume, gradually diminishes as we age.

Maintaining a healthy weight requires us to re-visit the body mass index (BMI) concept. Body weight in relationship to height, and the stability of that weight over time, are also factors used to determine the correct weight for a person. Either extreme obesity or being very thin is linked to potential increased health problems. Obese people experience increased heart disease, diabetes, and hypertension; while extremely thin people experience an increase in osteoporosis and early death. Throughout life, nutritional needs and number of calories change.

The modern way has fought the good fight against scurvy, rickets, pellagra, and goiter, only to lose the battle to overindulgence and malnutrition, from early childhood into old age. While we may grow old, we don't want to grow sick and fat. Yet, we all long for a "light in the tunnel" or a diet that can control weight and promote health without denying us the very pleasure of the food we eat. We need a new prescription that is designed for life-long health, not for short-term weight loss.

The fix? Eating more fruits, vegetables, legumes, whole grains, nuts, seeds, fiber, calcium, omega-3 fatty acids, and polyunsaturated fats. This should be coupled with eating less red meat, processed meat, sugar-sweetened beverages, and sodium. Dietary interventions really can alleviate morbidity. The best any of us can do is to make sure we stay active every day; get nutrients from food, not supplements; eat as many fruits, vegetables, and whole grains as possible daily; limit our intake of processed foods, salt, and meat of all kinds; and have a little fun every day. The longest-lived people in the world have been studied for years and these are their foundational tenets.

Bibliography

Reputable General Websites

Academy of Nutrition and Dietetics
www.eatright.org
Ad Fontes Media
www.adfontesmedia.com
Agency for Healthcare Research & Quality
www.ahrq.gov
American Cancer Society
www.cancer.org
American Council on Science and Health
www.acsh.org
American Diabetes Association
www.diabetes.org
American Heart Association
www.heart.org
American Journal of Clinical Nutrition
www.ajcn.org
American Medical Association
www.ama-assn.org
Animal Research Info
www.animalresearch.info
Big Think
www.bigthink.com
BioEthics Education Project
www.beep.ac.uk
Brookings Institution
www.brookings.edu/
Center for Reproductive Rights Retrieved
www.reproductiverights.org
Centers for Disease Control and
Prevention
www.cdc.gov
Cleveland Clinic
www.my.clevelandclinic.org/
Clinical Correlations
www.clinicalcorrelations.org
Cochrane
www.cochrane.org

The Conversation
www.theconversation.com/us
Fact Check.Org A Project of the
Annenberg Public Policy Center
www.factcheck.org
Go Ask Alice!
www.goaskalice.columbia.edu
Guttmacher Institute
www.guttmacher.org
Health on the Net
www.hon.ch
International Food Information Council
Foundation
www.foodinsight.org
Johns Hopkins Medicine
www.hopkinsmedicine.org
*Journal of the Academy of Nutrition and
Dietetics*
www.adajournal.org
Live Science
www.livescience.com
The Logic of Science
www.thelogicofscience.com
Mayo Clinic
www.mayoclinic.org
The Media Bias Chart
www.adfontesmedia.com
Medscape
www.medscape.com/today
Merck Manuals
www.merckmanuals.co
New England Journal of Medicine
www.nejm.org
Nutrition Reviews
www.academic.oup.com
Office of Dietary Supplements (ODS)
www.ods.nih.gov
The People's Pharmacy
www.peoplespharmacy.com

Pew Research Center
www.pewresearch.org
ProCon.org—Pros and Cons of
Controversial Issues
www.procon.org
ProPublica
www.propublica.org
PubMed—NCBI
www.ncbi.nlm.nih.gov
Quackwatch
www.quackwatch.org
Rand Corporation
www.rand.org
Reuters News Agency
www.reuters.com
Rewire News Group
www.rewirenewsgroup.com
Science News Magazine
www.sciencenews.org
Science-Based Medicine
www.sciencebasedmedicine.org
Snopes.com
www.snopes.com

The Straight Dope
www.straightdope.com
TheSkimm
www.theskimm.com
ThoughtCo
www.thoughtco.com
Union of Concerned Scientists
www.ucsusa.org
United States Department of Agriculture
(USDA)
www.usda.gov
United States Department of Health and
Human Services (HHS)
www.hhs.gov
United States Food and Drug
Administration (FDA)
www.fda.gov
United States General Services
Administration
www.gsa.gov
USAFacts
www.usafacts.org

Preface

National action plan to improve health literacy | health.gov. (n.d.). Retrieved from https://health.gov/our-work/health-literacy/national-action-plan-improve-health-literacy
Understanding literacy & numeracy | Health Literacy | CDC. (2019, November 13). https://www.cdc.gov/healthliteracy/learn/UnderstandingLiteracy.html

Chapter 1

Abdel-Hady, H., Nasef, N., Shabaan, A.E., & Nour, I. (2015). Caffeine therapy in preterm infants. *World Journal of Clinical Pediatrics*, *4*(4), 81–93. https://doi.org/10.5409/wjcp.v4.i4.81
About WIC-How WIC helps | USDA-FNS. (n.d.). Retrieved from https://www.fns.usda.gov/wic/about-wic-how-wic-helps
Adams, K.M., Lindell, K.C., Kohlmeier, M., & Zeisel, S.H. (2006). Status of nutrition education in medical schools. *The American Journal of Clinical Nutrition*, *83*(4), 941S-944S. https://doi.org/10.1093/ajcn/83.4.941S
Afshar, K., Stothers, L., Scott, H., & MacNeily, A.E. (2012). Cranberry juice for the prevention of pediatric urinary tract infection: A randomized controlled trial. *The Journal of Urology*, *188*(4 Suppl), 1584–1587. https://doi.org/10.1016/j.juro.2012.02.031
Afshin, A., Sur, P.J., Fay, K.A., Cornaby, L., Ferrara, G., Salama, J.S., … Murray, C.J.L. (2019). Health effects of dietary risks in 195 countries, 1990–2017: A systematic analysis for the Global Burden of Disease Study 2017. *The Lancet*, *0*(0). https://doi.org/10.1016/S0140-6736(19)30041-8
Ames, B.N., Shigenaga, M.K., & Hagen, T.M. (1993). Oxidants, antioxidants, and the degenerative diseases of aging. *Proceedings of the National Academy of Sciences of the United States of America*, *90*(17), 7915–7922. https://doi.org/10.1073/pnas.90.17.7915
Andrade, A.C., Cesena, F.H., Consolim-Colombo, F.M., Coimbra, S.R., Benjó, A.M., Krieger, E.M., & da Luz, P.L. (2009). Short-Term red wine consumption promotes differential effects on plasma levels of high-density lipoprotein cholesterol, sympathetic activity, and endothelial function in hypercholesterolemic, hypertensive, and

healthy subjects. *Clinics (Sao Paulo, Brazil)*, *64*(5), 435–442. https://doi.org/10.1590/S1807-59322009000500011

Avorn, J., Monane, M., Gurwitz, J.H., Glynn, R.J., Choodnovskiy, I., & Lipsitz, L.A. (1994). Reduction of bacteriuria and pyuria after ingestion of cranberry juice. *JAMA*, *271*(10), 751–754. https://doi.org/10.1001/jama.1994.03510340041031

Basu, A., Du, M., Leyva, M.J., Sanchez, K., Betts, N.M., Wu, M., ... Lyons, T.J. (2010). Blueberries decrease cardiovascular risk factors in obese men and women with metabolic syndrome. *The Journal of Nutrition*, *140*(9), 1582–1587. https://doi.org/10.3945/jn.110.124701

Blacker, B.C., Snyder, S.M., Eggett, D.L., & Parker, T.L. (2013). Consumption of blueberries with a high-carbohydrate, low-fat breakfast decreases postprandial serum markers of oxidation. *The British Journal of Nutrition*, *109*(9), 1670–1677. https://doi.org/10.1017/S0007114512003650

Brasure, M., MacDonald, R., Fuchs, E., Olson, C.M., Carlyle, M., Diem, S., ... Wilt, T.J. (2015). *Management of insomnia disorder*. Retrieved from http://www.ncbi.nlm.nih.gov/books/NBK343503/

A brief history of USDA food guides | ChooseMyPlate. (n.d.). Retrieved from https://www.choosemyplate.gov/eathealthy/brief-history-usda-food-guides

By the 2019 American Geriatrics Society Beers Criteria® Update Expert Panel. (2019). American Geriatrics Society 2019 updated AGS Beers Criteria® for potentially inappropriate medication use in older adults: 2019 AGS BEERS CRITERIA® UPDATE EXPERT PANEL. *Journal of the American Geriatrics Society*, *67*(4), 674–694. https://doi.org/10.1111/jgs.15767

Caffeine. (2009, July 26). Retrieved from https://web.archive.org/web/20090726194701/http://www.abc.net.au/quantum/poison/caffeine/caffeine.htm

Canada, H. (2018, October 4). Welcome to Canada's food guide. Retrieved from https://food-guide.canada.ca/en/, https://food-guide.canada.ca/

Cassidy, A., Mukamal, K.J., Liu, L., Franz, M., Eliassen, A.H., & Rimm, E.B. (2013). High anthocyanin intake is associated with a reduced risk of myocardial infarction in young and middle-aged women. *Circulation*, *127*(2), 188–196. https://doi.org/10.1161/CIRCULATIONAHA.112.122408

Chalons, P., Amor, S., Courtaut, F., Cantos-Villar, E., Richard, T., Auger, C., ... Delmas, D. (2018). Study of potential anti-inflammatory effects of red wine extract and resveratrol through a modulation of Interleukin-1-Beta in macrophages. *Nutrients*, *10*(12). https://doi.org/10.3390/nu10121856

Chamomile tea, will you help me sleep tonight? (n.d.). Retrieved from Office for Science and Society website: https://www.mcgill.ca/oss/article/health-and-nutrition/chamomile-tea-will-you-help-me-sleep-tonight

Chargé, S.B.P., & Rudnicki, M.A. (2004). Cellular and molecular regulation of muscle regeneration. *Physiological Reviews*, *84*(1), 209–238. https://doi.org/10.1152/physrev.00019.2003.

Consumer Health Digest: Trusted Source, Customer Reviews & Guides. (n.d.). Retrieved from https://www.consumerhealthdigest.com/

Cox, L., Williams, B., Sicherer, S., Oppenheimer, J., Sher, L., Hamilton, R., & Golden, D. (2008). Pearls and pitfalls of allergy diagnostic testing: Report from the American College of Allergy, Asthma and Immunology/American Academy of Allergy, Asthma and Immunology Specific IgE Test Task Force. *Annals of Allergy, Asthma & Immunology*, *101*(6), 580–592. https://doi.org/10.1016/S1081-1206(10)60220-7

Curcumin. (2014, April 28). Retrieved from Linus Pauling Institute website: https://lpi.oregonstate.edu/mic/dietary-factors/phytochemicals/curcumin

Devore, E.E., Kang, J.H., Breteler, M.M.B., & Grodstein, F. (2012). Dietary intakes of berries and flavonoids in relation to cognitive decline. *Annals of Neurology*, *72*(1), 135–143. https://doi.org/10.1002/ana.23594

Dhuley, J.N. (1999). Anti-oxidant effects of cinnamon (*Cinnamomum verum*) bark and greater cardamom (*Amomum subulatum*) seeds in rats fed high fat diet. *Indian Journal of Experimental Biology*, *37*(3), 238–242.

DoSomething.org. (n.d.). Retrieved from DoSomething.org website: https://www.dosomething.org/us/about/our-people

Eatright.org—Academy of Nutrition and Dietetics. (n.d.). Retrieved from https://www.eatright.org/

Falk, N., Cole, A., & Meredith, T.J. (2018). Evaluation of suspected dementia. *American Family Physician, 97*(6), 398–405. Retrieved from https://www.aafp.org/afp/2018/0315/p398.html

4 bears die of chocolate overdoses; expert proposes ban. (2019, June 24). Retrieved from https://web.archive.org/web/20190624173515/http://www.msn.com/en-us/news/us/4-bears-die-of-chocolate-overdoses-expert-proposes-ban/ar-AA8tCqh

Gracia-Sancho, J., & Salvadó, J. (eds.). (2017). *Gastrointestinal tissue: Oxidative stress and dietary antioxidants.* Elsevier/Academic Press, an imprint of Elsevier.

Greger, M. (n.d.). *Food industry-funded research bias | NutritionFacts.org.* Retrieved from https://nutritionfacts.org/video/food-industry-funded-research-bias/

Gunawardena, D., Karunaweera, N., Lee, S., van Der Kooy, F., Harman, D.G., Raju, R., … Münch, G. (2015). Anti-inflammatory activity of cinnamon (*C. zeylanicum* and *C. cassia*) extracts—Identification of E-cinnamaldehyde and o-methoxy cinnamaldehyde as the most potent bioactive compounds. *Food & Function, 6*(3), 910–919. https://doi.org/10.1039/c4fo00680a

Harvard T.H. Chan School of Public Health. Retrieved from Harvard T.H. Chan School of Public Health website: https://www.hsph.harvard.edu/

Haskell, C.F., Kennedy, D.O., Milne, A.L., Wesnes, K.A., & Scholey, A.B. (2008). The effects of L-theanine, caffeine and their combination on cognition and mood. *Biological Psychology, 77*(2), 113–122. https://doi.org/10.1016/j.biopsycho.2007.09.008

Hasler-Gehrer, S., Linecker, M., Keerl, A., Slieker, J., Descloux, A., Rosenberg, R., … Nocito, A. (2019). Does coffee intake reduce postoperative ileus after laparoscopic elective colorectal surgery? A prospective, randomized controlled study: The Coffee Study. *Diseases of the Colon and Rectum, 62*(8), 997–1004. https://doi.org/10.1097/DCR.0000000000001405

Holton, A.E., Gallagher, P.J., Ryan, C., Fahey, T., & Cousins, G. (2017). Consensus validation of the POSAMINO (POtentially Serious Alcohol–Medication INteractions in Older adults) criteria. *BMJ Open, 7*(11). https://doi.org/10.1136/bmjopen-2017-017453

Imhof, A., Woodward, M., Doering, A., Helbecque, N., Loewel, H., Amouyel, P., … Koenig, W. (2004). Overall alcohol intake, beer, wine, and systemic markers of inflammation in western Europe: Results from three MONICA samples (Augsburg, Glasgow, Lille). *European Heart Journal, 25*(23), 2092–2100. https://doi.org/10.1016/j.ehj.2004.09.032

Jarrett, C. (2017, July 26). Booty more amusing than ass, according to first in-depth study of the funniness of English words. Retrieved from Research Digest website: https://digest.bps.org.uk/2017/07/26/booty-more-amusing-than-ass-according-to-first-in-depth-study-of-the-funniness-of-english-words/

Jepson, R.G., & Craig, J.C. (2007). A systematic review of the evidence for cranberries and blueberries in UTI prevention. *Molecular Nutrition & Food Research, 51*(6), 738–745. https://doi.org/10.1002/mnfr.200600275

Jiménez-Monreal, A.M., García-Diz, L., Martínez-Tomé, M., Mariscal, M., & Murcia, M.A. (2009). Influence of cooking methods on antioxidant activity of vegetables. *Journal of Food Science, 74*(3), H97–H103. https://doi.org/10.1111/j.1750-3841.2009.01091.x

Kay, C.D., & Holub, B.J. (2002). The effect of wild blueberry (*Vaccinium angustifolium*) consumption on postprandial serum antioxidant status in human subjects. *The British Journal of Nutrition, 88*(4), 389–398. https://doi.org/10.1079/BJN2002665

Key findings about the online news landscape in America. *Pew Research Center.* Retrieved from https://www.pewresearch.org/fact-tank/2019/09/11/key-findings-about-the-online-news-landscape-in-america/

Kirkham, S., Akilen, R., Sharma, S., & Tsiami, A. (2009). The potential of cinnamon to reduce blood glucose levels in patients with type 2 diabetes and insulin resistance. *Diabetes, Obesity & Metabolism, 11*(12), 1100–1113. https://doi.org/10.1111/j.1463-1326.2009.01094.x

Korus, A., & Lisiewska, Z. (2011). Effect of preliminary processing and method of preservation on the content of selected antioxidative compounds in kale (*Brassica oleracea L.* var. Acephala) leaves. *Food Chemistry, 129*(1), 149–154. https://doi.org/10.1016/j.foodchem.2011.04.048

Krikorian, R., Shidler, M.D., Nash, T.A., Kalt, W., Vinqvist-Tymchuk, M.R., Shukitt-Hale, B., & Joseph, J.A. (2010). Blueberry supplementation improves memory in older adults. *Journal of Agricultural and Food Chemistry*, 58(7), 3996–4000. https://doi.org/10.1021/jf9029332

Latest news on hunger in US, Africa, Asia, global. (n.d.). Retrieved from World Hunger News website: https://www.worldhunger.org/

LAY'S® Classic Potato Chips. (n.d.). Retrieved from http://www.fritolay.com/snacks/product-page/lays/lays-classic-potato-chips

Lemonick, S. (n.d.). Everybody needs to stop with this turmeric molecule. Retrieved from https://www.forbes.com/sites/samlemonick/2017/01/19/everybody-needs-to-quit-it-with-this-turmeric-molecule/#7361107579ff

Liberale, L., Bonaventura, A., Montecucco, F., Dallegri, F., & Carbone, F. (2019). Impact of red wine consumption on cardiovascular health. *Current Medicinal Chemistry*, 26(19), 3542–3566. https://doi.org/10.2174/0929867324666170518100606

Maierean, S.M., Serban, M.C., Sahebkar, A., Ursoniu, S., Serban, A., Penson, P., ... Lipid and Blood Pressure Meta-analysis Collaboration (LBPMC) Group. (2017). The effects of cinnamon supplementation on blood lipid concentrations: A systematic review and meta-analysis. *Journal of Clinical Lipidology*, 11(6), 1393–1406. https://doi.org/10.1016/j.jacl.2017.08.004

Marton, R.M., Wang, X., Barabási, A.L., & Ioannidis, J.P.A. (2020). Science, advocacy, and quackery in nutritional books: An analysis of conflicting advice and purported claims of nutritional best-sellers. *Palgrave Communications*, 6(1), 1–6. https://doi.org/10.1057/s41599-020-0415-6

May 2021 keydata report | USDA-FNS. (n.d.). Retrieved from https://www.fns.usda.gov/data/may-2021-keydata-report

McKay, D.L., & Blumberg, J.B. (2006). A Review of the bioactivity and potential health benefits of chamomile tea (Matricaria recutita L.). *Phytotherapy Research*, 20(7), 519–530. https://doi.org/10.1002/ptr.1900

McManus, K.D. (2018, August 29). 10 superfoods to boost a healthy diet. Retrieved from Harvard Health Blog website: https://www.health.harvard.edu/blog/10-superfoods-to-boost-a-healthy-diet-2018082914463

Merck Manuals. The Trusted Provider of Medical Information since 1899. (n.d.). Retrieved from https://www.merckmanuals.com/

Moodie, R., Stuckler, D., Monteiro, C., Sheron, N., Neal, B., Thamarangsi, T., ... Casswell, S. (2013). Profits and pandemics: Prevention of harmful effects of tobacco, alcohol, and ultra-processed food and drink industries. *The Lancet*, 381(9867), 670–679. https://doi.org/10.1016/S0140-6736(12)62089-3

Moreno-Indias, I., Sánchez-Alcoholado, L., Pérez-Martínez, P., Andrés-Lacueva, C., Cardona, F., Tinahones, F., & Queipo-Ortuño, M.I. (2016). Red wine polyphenols modulate fecal microbiota and reduce markers of the metabolic syndrome in obese patients. *Food & Function*, 7(4), 1775–1787. https://doi.org/10.1039/c5fo00886g

The myth of IgG food panel testing | AAAAI. (n.d.). Retrieved from The American Academy of Allergy, Asthma & Immunology website: https://www.aaaai.org/conditions-and-treatments/library/allergy-library/IgG-food-test

Nelson, K.M., Dahlin, J.L., Bisson, J., Graham, J., Pauli, G.F., & Walters, M.A. (2017). The essential medicinal chemistry of curcumin. *Journal of Medicinal Chemistry*, 60(5), 1620–1637. https://doi.org/10.1021/acs.jmedchem.6b00975

Nestle, M. (2019). The Supplemental Nutrition Assistance Program (SNAP): History, politics, and public health implications. *American Journal of Public Health*, 109(12), 1631–1635. https://doi.org/10.2105/AJPH.2019.305361

Nutrition, C. for F.S. and A. (2019). How to understand and use the nutrition facts label. *FDA*. Retrieved from http://www.fda.gov/food/nutrition-education-resources-materials/how-understand-and-use-nutrition-facts-label

NutritionED.org. (n.d.). Retrieved from https://www.nutritioned.org/about.html

Nutrition.gov—Welcome. (n.d.). Retrieved from https://www.nutrition.gov/

Nylander, P.P.S. (1979). The Twinning Incidence in Nigeria. *Acta Geneticae Medicae et*

Gemellologiae: Twin Research, *28*(4), 261–263. https://doi.org/10.1017/S000156600000 8746

Osher Collaborative for Integrative Medicine. (n.d.). Retrieved from UCSF Osher Center for Integrative Medicine website: https://osher.ucsf.edu/osher-collaborative-integrative-medicine

Pahwa, R., & Jialal, I. (2019). Chronic inflammation. In *StatPearls*. Retrieved from http://www.ncbi.nlm.nih.gov/books/NBK493173/

Panche, A.N., Diwan, A.D., & Chandra, S.R. (2016). Flavonoids: An overview. *Journal of Nutritional Science*, *5*, e47. https://doi.org/10.1017/jns.2016.41

Pham, A.Q., Kourlas, H., & Pham, D.Q. (2007). Cinnamon supplementation in patients with type 2 diabetes mellitus. *Pharmacotherapy*, *27*(4), 595–599. https://doi.org/10.1592/phco.27.4.595

Ross, A.C. (ed.). (2014). *Modern nutrition in health and disease* (11th ed). Philadelphia: Wolters Kluwer Health/Lippincott Williams & Wilkins.

Staff, N.C.L. (n.d.). Olive oil mislabeling: Are consumers catching on? Retrieved from National Consumers League website: https://www.nclnet.org/evoo

States are using much-needed temporary flexibility in SNAP to respond to COVID-19 challenges. (n.d.). Center on Budget and Policy Priorities. Retrieved from https://www.cbpp.org/research/food-assistance/states-are-using-much-needed-temporary-flexibility-in-snap-to-respond-to

Stull, A.J., Cash, K.C., Johnson, W.D., Champagne, C.M., & Cefalu, W.T. (2010). Bioactives in blueberries improve insulin sensitivity in obese, insulin-resistant men and women. *The Journal of Nutrition*, *140*(10), 1764–1768. https://doi.org/10.3945/jn.110.125336

Vuong, T., Martineau, L.C., Ramassamy, C., Matar, C., & Haddad, P.S. (2007). Fermented Canadian lowbush blueberry juice stimulates glucose uptake and AMP-activated protein kinase in insulin-sensitive cultured muscle cells and adipocytes. *Canadian Journal of Physiology and Pharmacology*, *85*(9), 956–965. https://doi.org/10.1139/Y07–090

Webb, F.S., & Whitney, E.N. (2017). *Nutrition: concepts and controversies*.

Wilms, L.C., Boots, A.W., de Boer, V.C.J., Maas, L.M., Pachen, D.M.F.A., Gottschalk, R.W.H., … Kleinjans, J.C.S. (2007). Impact of multiple genetic polymorphisms on effects of a 4-week blueberry juice intervention on ex vivo induced lymphocytic DNA damage in human volunteers. *Carcinogenesis*, *28*(8), 1800–1806. https://doi.org/10.1093/carcin/bgm145

World Health Organization International. (n.d.). Retrieved from https://www.who.int

World hunger, poverty facts, statistics 2018. (n.d.). Retrieved from World Hunger News website: https://www.worldhunger.org/world-hunger-and-poverty-facts-and-statistics/

Chapter 2

Callaway, E. (2019). C-section babies are missing key microbes. *Nature*. https://doi.org/10.1038/d41586-019-02807-x

Cannon, B., & Nedergaard, J. (2008). Developmental biology: Neither fat nor flesh. *Nature*, *454*(7207), 947–948. https://doi.org/10.1038/454947a

Clawson, R.C., dela Cruz, L.N., Allen, S., Wolgemuth, T., Maner, A., Dorsett, A., & I'Anson, H. (2019). Continuous access to snacks from weaning onwards in female rats causes weight gain, insulin insensitivity, and sustained leptin resistance in adulthood. *Physiology & Behavior*, *201*, 165–174. https://doi.org/10.1016/j.physbeh.2018.11.026

Digitale, E. (n.d.). Antibody injection stops peanut allergy for 2 to 6 weeks, study shows. Retrieved from News Center website: http://med.stanford.edu/news/all-news/2019/11/antibody-injection-stops-peanut-allergy-for-2-to-6-weeks—study-.html

Faderl, M., Noti, M., Corazza, N., & Mueller, C. (2015). Keeping bugs in check: The mucus layer as a critical component in maintaining intestinal homeostasis. *IUBMB Life*, *67*(4), 275–285. https://doi.org/10.1002/iub.1374

Gilbert, J.A., Blaser, M.J., Caporaso, J.G., Jansson, J.K., Lynch, S.V., & Knight, R. (2018). Current understanding of the human microbiome. *Nature Medicine*, *24*(4), 392–400. https://doi.org/10.1038/nm.4517

Ma 02115 +1495-1000. (2017, August 16). The Microbiome. Retrieved from The Nutrition Source website: https://www.hsph.harvard.edu/nutritionsource/microbiome/

Makris, M.C., Alexandrou, A., Papatsoutsos, E.G., Malietzis, G., Tsilimigras, D.I., Guerron, A.D., & Moris, D. (2017). Ghrelin and obesity: Identifying gaps and dispelling myths. A reappraisal. *In Vivo (Athens, Greece)*, *31*(6), 1047–1050. https://doi.org/10.21873/invivo.11168

Marshall, B., & Adams, P.C. (2008). Helicobacter pylori—A Nobel pursuit? *Canadian Journal of Gastroenterology = Journal Canadien De Gastroenterologie*, *22*(11), 895–896. https://doi.org/10.1155/2008/459810

Maslowski, K.M., & Mackay, C.R. (2011). Diet, gut microbiota and immune responses. *Nature Immunology*, *12*(1), 5–9. https://doi.org/10.1038/ni0111-5

Mueller, N.T., Bakacs, E., Combellick, J., Grigoryan, Z., & Dominguez-Bello, M.G. (2015). The infant microbiome development: Mom matters. *Trends in Molecular Medicine*, *21*(2), 109–117. https://doi.org/10.1016/j.molmed.2014.12.002

Partrick, K.A., Chassaing, B., Beach, L.Q., McCann, K.E., Gewirtz, A.T., & Huhman, K.L. (2018). Acute and repeated exposure to social stress reduces gut microbiota diversity in Syrian hamsters. *Behavioural Brain Research*, *345*, 39–48. https://doi.org/10.1016/j.bbr.2018.02.005

Sears, C.L. (2005). A dynamic partnership: Celebrating our gut flora. *Anaerobe*, *11*(5), 247–251. https://doi.org/10.1016/j.anaerobe.2005.05.001

Sekirov, I., Russell, S.L., Antunes, L.C.M., & Finlay, B.B. (2010). Gut microbiota in health and disease. *Physiological Reviews*, *90*(3), 859–904. https://doi.org/10.1152/physrev.00045.2009

Shen, S., & Wong, C.H. (2016). Bugging inflammation: Role of the gut microbiota. *Clinical & Translational Immunology*, *5*(4), e72. https://doi.org/10.1038/cti.2016.12

Sicherer, S.H., & Sampson, H.A. (2014). Food allergy: Epidemiology, pathogenesis, diagnosis, and treatment. *Journal of Allergy and Clinical Immunology*, *133*(2), 291–307.e5. https://doi.org/10.1016/j.jaci.2013.11.020

Sommer, F., & Bäckhed, F. (2013). The gut microbiota—Masters of host development and physiology. *Nature Reviews. Microbiology*, *11*(4), 227–238. https://doi.org/10.1038/nrmicro2974

Willey, J.M., Sherwood, L., & Woolverton, C.J. (2014). *Prescott's microbiology* (Ninth edition). New York, NY: McGraw-Hill.

Yassour, M., Vatanen, T., Siljander, H., Hämäläinen, A.-M., Härkönen, T., Ryhänen, S.J., … Xavier, R.J. (2016). Natural history of the infant gut microbiome and impact of antibiotic treatment on bacterial strain diversity and stability. *Science Translational Medicine*, *8*(343), 343ra81. https://doi.org/10.1126/scitranslmed.aad0917

Zhu, X., Han, Y., Du, J., Liu, R., Jin, K., & Yi, W. (2017). Microbiota-gut-brain axis and the central nervous system. *Oncotarget*, *8*(32). https://doi.org/10.18632/oncotarget.17754s

Chapter 3

Bank, J., Teplica, D., & Keith, L. (2013). Important evidence for anatomic predetermination: The auto-mirroring phenomenon in skin. *Journal of the American Academy of Dermatology*, *68*(4), AB9. https://doi.org/10.1016/j.jaad.2012.12.040

Burgess, L. (n.d.). Waist-to-hip ratio: How does it affect your health? Retrieved from Medical News Today website: https://www.medicalnewstoday.com/articles/319439.php

Calculate your BMI—Standard BMI calculator. (n.d.). Retrieved from https://www.nhlbi.nih.gov/health/educational/lose_wt/BMI/bmicalc.htm

Chung, N., Park, M.-Y., Kim, J., Park, H.-Y., Hwang, H., Lee, C.-H., Han, J.-S., So, J., Park, J., & Lim, K. (2018). Non-exercise activity thermogenesis (NEAT): A component of total daily energy expenditure. *Journal of Exercise Nutrition & Biochemistry*, *22*(2), 23–30. https://doi.org/10.20463/jenb.2018.0013

Courcoulas, A.P., Yanovski, S.Z., Bonds, D., Eggerman, T.L., Horlick, M., Staten, M.A., & Arterburn, D.E. (2014). Long-term outcomes of bariatric surgery: A National Institutes of Health Symposium. *JAMA Surgery*, *149*(12), 1323. https://doi.org/10.1001/jamasurg.2014.2440

Fearon, K., Strasser, F., Anker, S.D., Bosaeus, I., Bruera, E., Fainsinger, R.L., ... Baracos, V.E. (2011). Definition and classification of cancer cachexia: An international consensus. *The Lancet Oncology*, 12(5), 489–495. https://doi.org/10.1016/S1470-2045(10)70218-7

Harvard Health. (n.d.). *Calorie counting made easy*. Harvard Health. Retrieved from https://www.health.harvard.edu/staying-healthy/calorie-counting-made-easy

Hawton, K., Norris, T., Crawley, E., & Hamilton-Shield, J. (2016). Is abuse associated with adolescent overweight and obesity?: A population cohort study. *Endocrine Abstracts*. https://doi.org/10.1530/endoabs.45.OC8.6

Jackson, A.S., Stanforth, P.R., Gagnon, J., Rankinen, T., Leon, A.S., Rao, D.C., Skinner, J.S., Bouchard, C., & Wilmore, J.H. (2002). The effect of sex, age and race on estimating percentage body fat from body mass index: The Heritage Family Study. *International Journal of Obesity*, 26(6), 789–796. https://doi.org/10.1038/sj.ijo.0802006

John, S., & Hoegerl, C. (2009). Nutritional deficiencies after gastric bypass surgery. *The Journal of the American Osteopathic Association*, 109(11), 601–604. https://doi.org/10.7556/jaoa.2009.109.11.601

NIMH » Eating Disorders. (n.d.). Retrieved from https://www.nimh.nih.gov/health/topics/eating-disorders/index.shtml

Peltzer, K., Pengpid, S., Samuels, T., Özcan, N., Mantilla, C., Rahamefy, O., Wong, M., & Gasparishvili, A. (2014). Prevalence of overweight/obesity and its associated factors among university students from 22 countries. *International Journal of Environmental Research and Public Health*, 11(7), 7425–7441. https://doi.org/10.3390/ijerph110707425

Ross, A.C. (ed.). (2014). *Modern nutrition in health and disease* (11th ed). Philadelphia: Wolters Kluwer Health/Lippincott Williams & Wilkins.

Sacks, F.M., Bray, G.A., Carey, V.J., Smith, S.R., Ryan, D.H., Anton, S.D., McManus, K., Champagne, C.M., Bishop, L.M., Laranjo, N., Leboff, M.S., Rood, J.C., de Jonge, L., Greenway, F.L., Loria, C.M., Obarzanek, E., & Williamson, D.A. (2009). Comparison of weight-loss diets with different compositions of fat, protein, and carbohydrates. *New England Journal of Medicine*, 360(9), 859–873. https://doi.org/10.1056/NEJMoa0804748

There are six different types of obesity, study argues. (2018, October 3). NHS.UK. https://www.nhs.uk/news/obesity/there-are-six-different-types-of-obesity-study-argues/

Types of bariatric surgery | *NIDDK*. (n.d.). National Institute of Diabetes and Digestive and Kidney Diseases. Retrieved from https://www.niddk.nih.gov/health-information/weight-management/bariatric-surgery/types

Udo, T., & Grilo, C.M. (2016). Perceived weight discrimination, childhood maltreatment, and weight gain in U.S. adults with overweight/obesity: Weight Discrimination, Childhood Adversity, and Weight. *Obesity*, 24(6), 1366–1372. https://doi.org/10.1002/oby.21474

Chapter 4

Allen, L.H., & Caballero, B. (2013). *Encyclopedia of human nutrition (3rd ed)*. Amsterdam: Elsevier.

A1C [Text]. (n.d.). Retrieved from https://medlineplus.gov/a1c.html

Artificial sweeteners and cancer [CgvArticle]. (2005, August 18). Retrieved from National Cancer Institute website: https://www.cancer.gov/about-cancer/causes-prevention/risk/diet/artificial-sweeteners-fact-sheet

Azad, M.B., Abou-Setta, A.M., Chauhan, B.F., Rabbani, R., Lys, J., Copstein, L., ... Zarychanski, R. (2017). Nonnutritive sweeteners and cardiometabolic health: A systematic review and meta-analysis of randomized controlled trials and prospective cohort studies. *CMAJ: Canadian Medical Association Journal = Journal de l'Association Medicale Canadienne*, 189(28), E929–E939. https://doi.org/10.1503/cmaj.161390

CFR—Code of Federal Regulations Title 21. (n.d.). Retrieved from https://www.accessdata.fda.gov/scripts/cdrh/cfdocs/cfcfr/CFRSearch.cfm?fr=172.804

Choose your carbs wisely. (n.d.). Retrieved from Mayo Clinic website: https://www.mayoclinic.org/healthy-lifestyle/nutrition-and-healthy-eating/in-depth/carbohydrates/art-20045705

Cornier, M.-A., Dabelea, D., Hernandez, T.L., Lindstrom, R.C., Steig, A.J., Stob, N.R., ...

Eckel, R.H. (2008). The Metabolic Syndrome. *Endocrine Reviews, 29*(7), 777–822. https://doi.org/10.1210/er.2008-0024

Donovan, P.J., & McIntyre, H.D. (2010). Drugs for gestational diabetes. *Australian Prescriber, 33*(5), 141–144. https://doi.org/10.18773/austprescr.2010.066

Dżugan, M., Tomczyk, M., Sowa, P., & Grabek-Lejko, D. (2018). Antioxidant activity as biomarker of honey variety. *Molecules (Basel, Switzerland), 23*(8). https://doi.org/10.3390/molecules23082069

Erejuwa, O.O., Sulaiman, S.A., Wahab, M.S.A., Sirajudeen, K.N.S., Salleh, S., & Gurtu, S. (2011). Differential responses to blood pressure and oxidative stress in streptozotocin-induced diabetic Wistar-Kyoto rats and spontaneously hypertensive rats: Effects of antioxidant (honey) treatment. *International Journal of Molecular Sciences, 12*(3), 1888–1907. https://doi.org/10.3390/ijms12031888

Erejuwa, O.O., Sulaiman, S.A., Wahab, M.S.A, Sirajudeen, K.N.S., Salleh, S., & Gurtu, S. (2012). Honey supplementation in spontaneously hypertensive rats elicits antihypertensive effect via amelioration of renal oxidative stress. *Oxidative Medicine and Cellular Longevity, 2012*, 1–14. https://doi.org/10.1155/2012/374037

Fructose and gout: What's the link? (2016, February 15). *Gout.* http://blog.arthritis.org/gout/fructose-sugar-gout/

Gheldof, N., Wang, X.-H., & Engeseth, N.J. (2002). Identification and quantification of antioxidant components of honeys from various floral sources. *Journal of Agricultural and Food Chemistry, 50*(21), 5870–5877. https://doi.org/10.1021/jf0256135

Global zero-calorie sweetener market projected to be worth USD 2.84 billion by 2021: Technavio | Business Wire. (n.d.). Retrieved from https://web.archive.org/web/20190328081134/https://www.businesswire.com/news/home/20170331005203/en/

Glycemic index and diabetes | ADA. (n.d.). Retrieved from https://www.diabetes.org/glycemic-index-and-diabetes

Grinstein, J.D. (2018, December 5). A new connection between the gut and the brain. *Scientific American.*

Jenkins, D.J., Wolever, T.M., Taylor, R.H., Barker, H., Fielden, H., Baldwin, J.M., … Goff, D.V. (1981). Glycemic index of foods: A physiological basis for carbohydrate exchange. *The American Journal of Clinical Nutrition, 34*(3), 362–366. https://doi.org/10.1093/ajcn/34.3.362

Kossoff, E.H., Zupec-Kania, B.A., Auvin, S., Ballaban-Gil, K.R., Christina Bergqvist, A.G., Blackford, R., … the Practice Committee of the Child Neurology Society. (2018). Optimal clinical management of children receiving dietary therapies for epilepsy: Updated recommendations of the International Ketogenic Diet Study Group. *Epilepsia Open, 3*(2), 175–192. https://doi.org/10.1002/epi4.12225

Kowalski, P. (n.d.). Myth: Too much sugar causes hyperactivity in children. Retrieved from Association for Psychological Science—APS website: https://www.psychologicalscience.org/uncategorized/myth-too-much-sugar-causes-hyperactivity-in-children.html

Kuzma, J.N., Cromer, G., Hagman, D.K., Breymeyer, K.L., Roth, C.L., Foster-Schubert, K.E., … Kratz, M. (2019). Consuming glucose-sweetened, not fructose-sweetened, beverages increases fasting insulin in healthy humans. *European Journal of Clinical Nutrition, 73*(3), 487–490. https://doi.org/10.1038/s41430-018-0297-5

Martini, F., Ober, W., Nath, J., Bartholomew, E., & Petti, K. (2018). *Visual anatomy & physiology* (3rd edition). NY, NY: Pearson.

Misra, H., Soni, M., Silawat, N., Mehta, D., Mehta, B.K., & Jain, D.C. (2011). Antidiabetic activity of medium-polar extract from the leaves of *Stevia rebaudiana* Bert. (Bertoni) on alloxan-induced diabetic rats. *Journal of Pharmacy & Bioallied Sciences, 3*(2), 242–248. https://doi.org/10.4103/0975-7406.80779

Mitchell, H. (ed.). (2006). *Sweeteners and sugar alternatives in food technology.* Oxford ; Ames, Iowa: Blackwell Pub.

National Center for Biotechnology Information. PubChem Database. Phenylalanine, CID=6140, https://pubchem.ncbi.nlm.nih.gov/compound/Phenylalanine

Nicklas, T.A., Qu, H., Hughes, S.O., Wagner, S.E., Foushee, H.R., & Shewchuk, R.M. (2009). Prevalence of self-reported lactose intolerance in a multiethnic sample of adults: *Nutrition Today, 44*(5), 222–227. https://doi.org/10.1097/NT.0b013e3181b9caa6

Nutrition, C. for F. S. and A. (2019, September 6). Generally Recognized as Safe (GRAS). Retrieved from FDA website: http://www.fda.gov/food/food-ingredients-packaging/generally-recognized-safe-gras

Oliveira, R. (2015, May 14). Discover the surprising truth about the GI. Retrieved from UC Davis Integrative Medicine website: https://ucdintegrativemedicine.com/2015/05/discover-the-s-h-about-the-gi/

Paleo diet: Eat like a cave man and lose weight? (n.d.). Retrieved from Mayo Clinic website: https://www.mayoclinic.org/healthy-lifestyle/nutrition-and-healthy-eating/in-depth/paleo-diet/art-20111182

Roberts, J. (2015, December 8). Sickening sweet. Retrieved from Science History Institute website: https://www.sciencehistory.org/distillations/sickening-sweet

Stevia herb shakes up global sweetener market | The Independent. (n.d.). Retrieved from https://www.independent.co.uk/life-style/health-and-families/stevia-herb-shakes-up-global-sweetener-market-5531238.html

Sugar 101. (n.d.). Retrieved from www.heart.org website: https://www.heart.org/en/healthy-living/healthy-eating/eat-smart/sugar/sugar-101

Weber, D.D., Aminazdeh-Gohari, S., & Kofler, B. (2018). Ketogenic diet in cancer therapy. *Aging, 10*(2), 164–165. https://doi.org/10.18632/aging.101382

Weihrauch, M.R., & Diehl, V. (2004). Artificial sweeteners—Do they bear a carcinogenic risk? *Annals of Oncology, 15*(10), 1460–1465. https://doi.org/10.1093/annonc/mdh256

Which is more effective, Beano or Gas-X for gas from ulcerative colitis? (n.d.). Retrieved from Drugs.com website: https://www.drugs.com/medical-answers/effective-beano-gas-1138864/

Wolraich, M.L. (1995). The effect of sugar on behavior or cognition in children: A meta-analysis. *JAMA, 274*(20), 1617. https://doi.org/10.1001/jama.1995.03530200053037

Xylitol uses, benefits & dosage—Drugs.com Herbal Database. (n.d.). Retrieved from Drugs.com website: https://www.drugs.com/npp/xylitol.html

Yaghoobi, N., Al-Waili, N., Ghayour-Mobarhan, M., Parizadeh, S.M.R., Abasalti, Z., Yaghoobi, Z., … Ferns, G.A.A. (2008). Natural honey and cardiovascular risk factors; Effects on blood glucose, cholesterol, triacylglycerole, CRP, and body weight compared with sucrose. *The Scientific World JOURNAL, 8*, 463–469. https://doi.org/10.1100/tsw.2008.64

Yang, Q., Zhang, Z., Gregg, E.W., Flanders, W.D., Merritt, R., & Hu, F.B. (2014). Added sugar intake and cardiovascular diseases mortality among US adults. *JAMA Internal Medicine, 174*(4), 516. https://doi.org/10.1001/jamainternmed.2013.13563

Yoquinto, L., & Health, 2013. (n.d.). The truth about aspartame. Retrieved from Livescience.com website: https://www.livescience.com/36257-aspartame-health-effects-artificial-sweetener.html

Chapter 5

CDC. (2018, September 7). Cholesterol screenings. Retrieved from Centers for Disease Control and Prevention website: https://www.cdc.gov/features/cholesterol-screenings/index.html

Cholesterol levels: MedlinePlus lab test information. (n.d.). Retrieved from https://medlineplus.gov/lab-tests/cholesterol-levels/

DuBroff, R., Malhotra, A., & de Lorgeril, M. (2020). Hit or miss: The new cholesterol targets. *BMJ Evidence-Based Medicine*, bmjebm-2020–111413. https://doi.org/10.1136/bmjebm-2020–111413

Durham, S. (n.d.). *USDA ARS online magazine going nuts over calories*. Retrieved from https://agresearchmag.ars.usda.gov/2018/mar/calories/#printdiv

Eschner, K. (n.d.). The 1870s dairy lobby turned margarine pink so people would buy butter. Retrieved from Smithsonian website: https://www.smithsonianmag.com/smart-news/1870s-dairy-lobby-turned-margarine-pink-so-people-would-buy-butter-180963328/

Facts about monounsaturated fats: MedlinePlus Medical Encyclopedia. (n.d.). Retrieved from https://medlineplus.gov/ency/patientinstructions/000785.htm

Félix-Redondo, F.J., Grau, M., & Fernández-Bergés, D. (2013). Cholesterol and cardiovascular disease in the elderly. Facts and gaps. *Aging and Disease, 4*(3), 154–169.

Fish oil and omega-3 and -7 supplements review (Including krill, algal, calamari, and sea buckthorn oil supplements). (n.d.). Retrieved from ConsumerLab.com website: /reviews/fish_oil_supplements_review/omega3/

Gardner, C.D., Kiazand, A., Alhassan, S., Kim, S., Stafford, R.S., Balise, R.R., … King, A.C. (2007). Comparison of the Atkins, Zone, Ornish, and LEARN diets for change in weight and related risk factors among overweight premenopausal women: The A TO Z Weight Loss Study: A randomized trial. *JAMA, 297*(9), 969. https://doi.org/10.1001/jama.297.9.969

Gioxari, A., Kaliora, A.C., Marantidou, F., & Panagiotakos, D.P. (2018). Intake of ω-3 poly-unsaturated fatty acids in patients with rheumatoid arthritis: A systematic review and meta-analysis. *Nutrition (Burbank, Los Angeles County, Calif.), 45*, 114–124.e4. https://doi.org/10.1016/j.nut.2017.06.023

Guasch-Ferré, M., Liu, X., Malik, V.S., Sun, Q., Willett, W.C., Manson, J.E., … Bhupathiraju, S.N. (2017). Nut consumption and risk of cardiovascular disease. *Journal of the American College of Cardiology, 70*(20), 2519–2532. https://doi.org/10.1016/j.jacc.2017.09.035

How many eggs can you eat on a heart-healthy diet? (2019, July 18). Retrieved from Health Essentials from Cleveland Clinic website: https://health.clevelandclinic.org/how-many-eggs-can-you-eat-on-a-heart-healthy-diet/

Hu, Y., Hu, F.B., & Manson, J.E. (2019). Marine omega-3 supplementation and cardiovascular disease: An updated meta-analysis of 13 randomized controlled trials involving 127,477 participants. *Journal of the American Heart Association: Cardiovascular and Cerebrovascular Disease, 8*(19). https://doi.org/10.1161/JAHA.119.013543

Kristensen, M.L., Christensen, P.M., & Hallas, J. (2015). The effect of statins on average survival in randomised trials, an analysis of end point postponement: Table 1. *BMJ Open, 5*(9), e007118. https://doi.org/10.1136/bmjopen-2014–007118

Kühn, J., Schutkowski, A., Kluge, H., Hirche, F., & Stangl, G.I. (2014). Free-range farming: A natural alternative to produce vitamin D-enriched eggs. *Nutrition (Burbank, Los Angeles County, Calif.), 30*(4), 481–484. https://doi.org/10.1016/j.nut.2013.10.002

Kyolic Aged Garlic Extract. (n.d.). Retrieved from https://kyolic.com/about-us/

Lee, Y., Berryman, C.E., West, S.G., Chen, C.-Y.O., Blumberg, J.B., Lapsley, K.G., … Kris-Etherton, P.M. (2017). Effects of dark chocolate and almonds on cardiovascular risk factors in overweight and obese individuals: A randomized controlled-feeding trial. *Journal of the American Heart Association, 6*(12). https://doi.org/10.1161/JAHA.116.005162

Li, X., Bi, X., Wang, S., Zhang, Z., Li, F., & Zhao, A.Z. (2019). Therapeutic potential of ω-3 polyunsaturated fatty acids in human autoimmune diseases. *Frontiers in Immunology, 10*. https://doi.org/10.3389/fimmu.2019.02241

Liu, G., Guasch-Ferre, M., Hu, Y., Li, Y., Hu, F.B., Rimm, E.B., … Sun, Q. (2019). Nut consumption in relation to cardiovascular disease incidence and mortality among patients with diabetes mellitus. *Circulation Research.* https://doi.org/10.1161/CIRCRESAHA.118.314316

Matthews, D. (2015, December 25). Cage-free, free range, organic: What all those egg labels really mean. Retrieved from Vox website: https://www.vox.com/2015/12/25/10662742/egg-labels-cage-free

McGill, H.C., McMahan, C.A., & Gidding, S.S. (2008). Preventing heart disease in the 21st century: Implications of the Pathobiological Determinants of Atherosclerosis in Youth (PDAY) study. *Circulation, 117*(9), 1216–1227. https://doi.org/10.1161/CIRCULATIONAHA.107.717033

Mendis, S., Puska, P., Norrving, B., World Health Organization, World Heart Federation, & World Stroke Organization (Eds.). (2011). *Global atlas on cardiovascular disease prevention and control.* Geneva: World Health Organization in collaboration with the World Heart Federation and the World Stroke Organization.

Molina-Leyva, I., Molina-Leyva, A., & Bueno-Cavanillas, A. (2017). Efficacy of nutritional supplementation with omega-3 and omega-6 fatty acids in dry eye syndrome: A systematic review of randomized clinical trials. *Acta Ophthalmologica, 95*(8), e677–e685. https://doi.org/10.1111/aos.13428

Norwood, F.B., & Lusk, J. (2011). *Compassion, by the pound: The economics of farm animal welfare.* New York: Oxford University Press.

O'Donnell, M.J., Chin, S.L., Rangarajan, S., Xavier, D., Liu, L., Zhang, H., … INTERSTROKE investigators. (2016). Global and regional effects of potentially modifiable risk factors associated with acute stroke in 32 countries (INTERSTROKE): A case-control study. *Lancet (London, England)*, *388*(10046), 761–775. https://doi.org/10.1016/S0140-6736(16)30506-2

O'Keefe, E.L., Harris, W.S., DiNicolantonio, J.J., Elagizi, A., Milani, R.V., Lavie, C.J., & O'Keefe, J.H. (2019). Sea change for marine omega-3s: Randomized trials show fish oil reduces cardiovascular events. *Mayo Clinic Proceedings*. https://doi.org/10.1016/j.mayocp.2019.04.027

President's Council on Sports, F. & N. (2012, July 20). Dietary guidelines for Americans [Text]. Retrieved from HHS.gov website: https://www.hhs.gov/fitness/eat-healthy/dietary-guidelines-for-americans/index.html *2015–2020 Dietary Guidelines for Americans*. (n.d.). 144.

Ried, K., Travica, N., & Sali, A. (2018). The effect of kyolic aged garlic extract on gut microbiota, inflammation, and cardiovascular markers in hypertensives: The GarGIC Trial. *Frontiers in Nutrition*, *5*, 122. https://doi.org/10.3389/fnut.2018.00122

Rodrigues, C., & Percival, S.S. (2019). Immunomodulatory effects of glutathione, garlic derivatives, and hydrogen sulfide. *Nutrients*, *11*(2). https://doi.org/10.3390/nu11020295

Soltani, S., Chitsazi, M.J., & Salehi-Abargouei, A. (2018). The effect of dietary approaches to stop hypertension (DASH) on serum inflammatory markers: A systematic review and meta-analysis of randomized trials. *Clinical Nutrition*, *37*(2), 542–550. https://doi.org/10.1016/j.clnu.2017.02.018

Terés, S., Barceló-Coblijn, G., Benet, M., Álvarez, R., Bressani, R., Halver, J.E., & Escribá, P.V. (2008). Oleic acid content is responsible for the reduction in blood pressure induced by olive oil. *Proceedings of the National Academy of Sciences*, *105*(37), 13811–13816. https://doi.org/10.1073/pnas.0807500105

Zhu, Y., Anand, R., Geng, X., & Ding, Y. (2018). A mini review: Garlic extract and vascular diseases. *Neurological Research*, *40*(6), 421–425. https://doi.org/10.1080/01616412.2018.1451269

Chapter 6

About Us. (n.d.). Retrieved from Meatless Monday website: https://www.meatlessmonday.com/about-us/

Abuse, N. I. on D. (n.d.). What are the side effects of anabolic steroid misuse? Retrieved from https://www.drugabuse.gov/publications/research-reports/steroids-other-appearance-performance-enhancing-drugs-apeds/what-are-side-effects-anabolic-steroid-misuse

Anfinsen, C.B., Edsall, J.T., & Richards, F.M. (1972). *Advances in protein chemistry*. New York: Academic Press.

Animal feeding operations | NRCS. (n.d.). Retrieved from https://www.nrcs.usda.gov/wps/portal/nrcs/main/national/plantsanimals/livestock/afo/

BDA releases top 5 celeb diets to avoid in 2019. (n.d.). Retrieved from https://www.bda.uk.com/news/view?id=224

Bronson, F.H., & Matherne, C.M. (1997). Exposure to anabolic-androgenic steroids shortens life span of male mice. *Medicine and Science in Sports and Exercise*, *29*(5), 615–619. https://doi.org/10.1097/00005768-199705000-00005

Budhathoki, S., Sawada, N., Iwasaki, M., Yamaji, T., Goto, A., Kotemori, A., ... Japan Public Health Center–based Prospective Study Group. (2019). Association of animal and plant protein intake with all-cause and cause-specific mortality. *JAMA Internal Medicine*. https://doi.org/10.1001/jamainternmed.2019.2806

Canned tuna and salmon reviews and information. (n.d.). Retrieved from ConsumerLab.com website: /reviews/canned-tuna-and-salmon-review/canned-tuna-and-salmon/

CIS Index to Presidential Executive Orders & Proclamations: Apr. 30, 1789 to Mar. 4, 1921, George Washington to Woodrow Wilson. 10 v. (1986). Congressional Information Service, Incorporated.

D'Adamo, P., Whitney, C., & D'Adamo, P. (2002). *Complete blood type encyclopedia: The A-Z reference guide for the blood type connection to symptoms, disease, conditions, vitamins, supplements, herbs, and food*. New York: Riverhead Books.

Davis, C., Bryan, J., Hodgson, J., & Murphy, K. (2015). Definition of the Mediterranean Diet; A literature review. *Nutrients*, *7*(11), 9139–9153. https://doi.org/10.3390/nu7115459

Dioguardi, F.S. (2011). Clinical use of amino acids as dietary supplement: Pros and cons. *Journal of Cachexia, Sarcopenia and Muscle*, 2(2), 75–80. https://doi.org/10.1007/s13539-011-0032-8

Doerge, D.R., & Sheehan, D.M. (2002). Goitrogenic and estrogenic activity of soy isoflavones. *Environmental Health Perspectives*, 110 Suppl 3, 349–353. https://doi.org/10.1289/ehp.02110s3349

Everts, S. (2012). The Maillard Reaction turns 100. *Chemical & Engineering News Archive*, 90(40), 58–60. https://doi.org/10.1021/cen-09040-scitech2

Flail, G.J. (2011). Why *"flexitarian" was a word of the year: carno-phallogocentrism and the lexicon of vegetable-based diets*.

Foley, J.A., Ramankutty, N., Brauman, K.A., Cassidy, E.S., Gerber, J.S., Johnston, M., … Zaks, D.P.M. (2011). Solutions for a cultivated planet. *Nature*, 478(7369), 337–342. https://doi.org/10.1038/nature10452

Food Safety and Inspection Service. (n.d.). Retrieved from https://www.fsis.usda.gov/wps/wcm/connect/fsis-content/internet/main/topics/food-safety-education/get-answers/food-safety-fact-sheets/production-and-inspection/fsis-further-strengthens-protections-against-bovine-spongiform-encephalopathy-bse/fsis-further-strengthens-protections-against-bse

Gerber, P.J., & Food and Agriculture Organization of the United Nations (Eds.). (2013). *Tackling climate change through livestock: A global assessment of emissions and mitigation opportunities*. Rome: Food and Agriculture Organization of the United Nations.

Gilchrist Mary J., Greko Christina, Wallinga David B., Beran George W., Riley David G., & Thorne Peter S. (2007). The potential role of concentrated animal feeding operations in infectious disease epidemics and antibiotic resistance. *Environmental Health Perspectives*, 115(2), 313–316. https://doi.org/10.1289/ehp.8837

Gundry, S.R., & Buehl, O.B. (2017). *The plant paradox: The hidden dangers in "healthy" foods that cause disease and weight gain* (First edition). New York, NY: Harper Wave, an imprint of HarperCollins Publishers.

Hodge, J. E. (1953). Dehydrated foods, chemistry of browning reactions in model systems. *Journal of Agricultural and Food Chemistry*, 1(15), 928–943. https://doi.org/10.1021/jf60015a004

Humes, M. (2009, November 23). The way we ate: The year Harry Truman passed on pumpkin pie. Retrieved from Diner's Journal Blog website: https://dinersjournal.blogs.nytimes.com/2009/11/23/the-way-we-ate-the-year-harry-truman-passed-on-pumpkin-pie/

Johnston, C.S., Day, C.S., & Swan, P.D. (2002). Postprandial thermogenesis is increased 100% on a high-protein, low-fat diet versus a high-carbohydrate, low-fat diet in healthy, young women. *Journal of the American College of Nutrition*, 21(1), 55–61. https://doi.org/10.1080/07315724.2002.10719194

Keen, B., & Haynes, K. (2009). *A history of Latin America*. Boston: Houghton Mifflin Harcourt.

Levinovitz, A. (n.d.). What if your gluten intolerance is all in your head? Retrieved from New Scientist website: https://www.newscientist.com/article/dn23851-what-if-your-gluten-intolerance-is-all-in-your-head/Lopatto, E., Choi, J., Colina, A., Ma, L., Howe, A., & Hinsa-Leasure, S. (2019). Characterizing the soil microbiome and quantifying antibiotic resistance gene dynamics in agricultural soil following swine CAFO manure application. *PLoS ONE*, 14(8). https://doi.org/10.1371/journal.pone.0220770

Medicine, C. for V. (2019). Steroid hormone implants used for growth in food-producing animals. *FDA*. Retrieved from http://www.fda.gov/animal-veterinary/product-safety-information/steroid-hormone-implants-used-growth-food-producing-animals

Mercury and health. (n.d.). Retrieved from https://www.who.int/news-room/fact-sheets/detail/mercury-and-health

Morais, J.A., Chevalier, S., & Gougeon, R. (2006). Protein turnover and requirements in the healthy and frail elderly. *The Journal of Nutrition, Health & Aging*, 10(4), 272–283.

Mottram, D.S., Wedzicha, B.L., & Dodson, A.T. (2002). Acrylamide is formed in the Maillard reaction. *Nature*, 419(6906), 448–449. https://doi.org/10.1038/419448a

Ohara, T., Sato, T., Shimizu, N., Prescher, G., Schwind, H., Weiberg, O., … Greim, H. (2011). Acrylic acid and derivatives. In Wiley-VCH Verlag GmbH & Co. KGaA (Ed.), *Ullmann's*

Encyclopedia of Industrial Chemistry (p. a01_161.pub3). https://doi.org/10.1002/14356007. a01_161.pub3

Qian, F., Liu, G., Hu, F.B., Bhupathiraju, S.N., & Sun, Q. (2019). Association between plant-based dietary patterns and risk of type 2 diabetes: A systematic review and meta-analysis. *JAMA Internal Medicine.* https://doi.org/10.1001/jamainternmed.2019.2195

Sathyapalan, T., Köhrle, J., Rijntjes, E., Rigby, A.S., Dargham, S.R., Kilpatrick, E.S., & Atkin, S.L. (2018). The effect of high dose isoflavone supplementation on serum reverse T3 in euthyroid men with type 2 diabetes and post-menopausal women. *Frontiers in Endocrinology, 9.* https://doi.org/10.3389/fendo.2018.00698

Satija, A., Bhupathiraju, S.N., Rimm, E.B., Spiegelman, D., Chiuve, S.E., Borgi, L., ... Hu, F.B. (2016). plant-based dietary patterns and incidence of type 2 diabetes in U.S. men and women: results from three prospective cohort studies. *PLoS Medicine, 13*(6), e1002039. https://doi.org/10.1371/journal.pmed.1002039

Satija, A., Bhupathiraju, S.N., Spiegelman, D., Chiuve, S.E., Manson, J.E., Willett, W., ... Hu, F.B. (2017). Healthful and unhealthful plant-based diets and the risk of coronary heart disease in U.S. adults. *Journal of the American College of Cardiology, 70*(4), 411–422. https://doi.org/10.1016/j.jacc.2017.05.047

Schlick, G., & Bubenheim, D.L. (1993). *Quinoa: An emerging new crop with potential for CELSS.* Retrieved from https://ntrs.nasa.gov/search.jsp?R=19940015664

Science of cooking—Science of food and cooking. (n.d.). Retrieved from https://www.scienceofcooking.com/

Sedighi, M., Bahmani, M., Asgary, S., Beyranvand, F., & Rafieian-Kopaei, M. (2017). A review of plant-based compounds and medicinal plants effective on atherosclerosis. *Journal of Research in Medical Sciences, 22*(1), 30. https://doi.org/10.4103/1735-1995.202151

Shai, I., Schwarzfuchs, D., Henkin, Y., Shahar, D.R., Witkow, S., Greenberg, I., ... Stampfer, M.J. (2008). Weight loss with a low-carbohydrate, Mediterranean, or low-fat Diet. *New England Journal of Medicine, 359*(3), 229–241. https://doi.org/10.1056/NEJMoa0708681

Shmerling, R.H. (2017, May 12). Diet not working? Maybe it's not your type. Retrieved November 5, 2019, from Harvard Health Blog website: https://www.health.harvard.edu/blog/diet-not-working-maybe-its-not-your-type-2017051211678

Supasyndh, O., Satirapoj, B., Aramwit, P., Viroonudomphol, D., Chaiprasert, A., Thanachatwej, V., ... Kopple, J.D. (2013). Effect of oral anabolic steroid on muscle strength and muscle growth in hemodialysis patients. *Clinical Journal of the American Society of Nephrology : CJASN, 8*(2), 271–279. https://doi.org/10.2215/CJN.00380112

U.S. EPA, O. (2015, August 25). Guidelines for eating fish that contain mercury [Overviews and Factsheets]. Retrieved from US EPA website: https://www.epa.gov/mercury/guidelines-eating-fish-contain-mercury

Vauquelin L.N., & Robiquet, P.J. (1806). The discovery of a new plant principle in Asparagus sativus. *Annales de Chimie, 57*: 88–93.

Veldhorst, M.A.B., Westerterp, K.R., van Vught, A.J.A.H., & Westerterp-Plantenga, M.S. (2010). Presence or absence of carbohydrates and the proportion of fat in a high-protein diet affect appetite suppression but not energy expenditure in normal-weight human subjects fed in energy balance. *The British Journal of Nutrition, 104*(9), 1395–1405. https://doi.org/10.1017/S0007114510002060

Veldhorst, M.A.B., Westerterp-Plantenga, M.S., & Westerterp, K.R. (2009). Gluconeogenesis and energy expenditure after a high-protein, carbohydrate-free diet. *The American Journal of Clinical Nutrition, 90*(3), 519–526. https://doi.org/10.3945/ajcn.2009.27834

Vickery, H.B., & Schmidt, C.L.A. (1931). The history of the discovery of the amino acids. *Chemical Reviews, 9*(2), 169–318. https://doi.org/10.1021/cr60033a001

Virk-Baker, M.K., Nagy, T.R., Barnes, S., & Groopman, J. (2014). Dietary acrylamide and human cancer: A systematic review of literature. *Nutrition and Cancer, 66*(5), 774–790. https://doi.org/10.1080/01635581.2014.916323

West, B.M., Liggit, P., Clemans, D.L., & Francoeur, S.N. (2011). Antibiotic resistance, gene transfer, and water quality patterns observed in waterways near CAFO farms and wastewater treatment facilities. *Water, Air, & Soil Pollution, 217*(1), 473–489. https://doi.org/10.1007/s11270-010-0602-y

Yaffe-Bellany, D. (2019, October 14). The new makers of plant-based meat? Big meat companies. *The New York Times*. Retrieved from https://www.nytimes.com/2019/10/14/business/the-new-makers-of-plant-based-meat-big-meat-companies.html

Chapter 7

Agathocleous, M., Meacham, C.E., Burgess, R.J., Piskounova, E., Zhao, Z., Crane, G.M., … Morrison, S.J. (2017). Ascorbate regulates haematopoietic stem cell function and leukaemogenesis. *Nature, 549*(7673), 476–481. https://doi.org/10.1038/nature23876

Allen, R.E., & Kirby, K.A. (2012). Nocturnal leg cramps. *American Family Physician, 86*(4), 350–355.

American Association of Poison Control Centers (AAPCC)—Annual Report. (n.d.). Retrieved from https://aapcc.org/annual-reports

Anderson, T.W., Reid, D.B., & Beaton, G.H. (1972). Vitamin C and the common cold: A double-blind trial. *Canadian Medical Association Journal, 107*(6), 503–508.

Barbarawi, M., Kheiri, B., Zayed, Y., Barbarawi, O., Dhillon, H., Swaid, B., … Manson, J.E. (2019). Vitamin D supplementation and cardiovascular disease risks in more than 83,000 individuals in 21 randomized clinical trials: A Meta-analysis. *JAMA Cardiology, 4*(8), 765–776. https://doi.org/10.1001/jamacardio.2019.1870

Biesalski, H.K. (2020). Vitamin D deficiency and co-morbidities in COVID-19 patients—A fatal relationship? *NFS Journal, 20*, 10–21. https://doi.org/10.1016/j.nfs.2020.06.001

Bogden, J.D., & Klevay, L.M. (2000). *Clinical nutrition of the essential trace elements and minerals: The guide for health professionals*. Retrieved from https://public.ebookcentral.proquest.com/choice/publicfullrecord.aspx?p=3086011

Burt, L.A., Billington, E.O., Rose, M.S., Raymond, D.A., Hanley, D.A., & Boyd, S.K. (2019). Effect of high-dose vitamin D supplementation on volumetric bone density and bone strength: A randomized clinical trial. *JAMA, 322*(8), 736. https://doi.org/10.1001/jama.2019.11889

Carr, A.C., & Maggini, S. (2017). Vitamin C and immune function. *Nutrients, 9*(11). https://doi.org/10.3390/nu9111211

Douglas, R.M., Hemila, H., D'Souza, R., Chalker, E.B., & Treacy, B. (2004). Vitamin C for preventing and treating the common cold. *The Cochrane Database of Systematic Reviews* (4), CD000980. https://doi.org/10.1002/14651858.CD000980.pub2

Exercise for your bone health | NIH Osteoporosis and Related Bone Diseases National Resource Center. (n.d.). Retrieved from https://www.bones.nih.gov/health-info/bone/bone-health/exercise/exercise-your-bone-health

Garrison, S.R., Allan, G.M., Sekhon, R.K., Musini, V.M., & Khan, K.M. (2012). Magnesium for skeletal muscle cramps. *The Cochrane Database of Systematic Reviews* (9), CD009402. https://doi.org/10.1002/14651858.CD009402.pub2

Gómez, E., Quidel, S., Bravo-Soto, G., & Ortigoza, Á. (2018). Does vitamin C prevent the common cold? *Medwave, 18*(4), e7235. https://doi.org/10.5867/medwave.2018.04.7236

Gummin, D.D., Mowry, J.B., Spyker, D.A., Brooks, D.E., Fraser, M.O., & Banner, W. (2017). 2016 Annual Report of the American Association of Poison Control Centers' National Poison Data System (NPDS): 34th Annual Report. *Clinical Toxicology, 55*(10), 1072–1254. https://doi.org/10.1080/15563650.2017.1388087

Harvard Health. (n.d.). Vitamin D and your health: Breaking old rules, raising new hopes. Retrieved from Harvard Health website: https://www.health.harvard.edu/staying-healthy/vitamin-d-and-your-health-breaking-old-rules-raising-new-hopes

Heaney, R.P. (2000). Calcium, dairy products and osteoporosis. *Journal of the American College of Nutrition, 19* (2 Suppl), 83S-99S. https://doi.org/10.1080/07315724.2000.10718088

Heaney, R.P. (n.d.). The roles of calcium and vitamin D in skeletal health: An evolutionary perspective. Retrieved from http://www.fao.org/3/W7336T/w7336t03.htm

Helmenstine, A.M., sciences, P. D. D. H. holds a P. D. in biomedical, Writer, I. a S., educator, school, consultant S. has taught science courses at the high, college, & Levels, G. (n.d.).

Which elements are in the human body? Retrieved from ThoughtCo website: https://www. thoughtco.com/elements-in-the-human-body-p2–602188

Hu, Z., Tao, S., Liu, H., Pan, G., Li, B., & Zhang, Z. (2019). The association between polymorphisms of vitamin D metabolic-related genes and vitamin D3 supplementation in type 2 diabetic patients. *Journal of Diabetes Research, 2019.* https://doi.org/10.1155/2019/8289741

Hunnicutt, J., He, K., & Xun, P. (2014). Dietary iron intake and body iron stores are associated with risk of coronary heart disease in a meta-analysis of prospective cohort studies. *The Journal of Nutrition, 144*(3), 359–366. https://doi.org/10.3945/jn.113.185124

Hurrell, R., & Egli, I. (2010). Iron bioavailability and dietary reference values. *The American Journal of Clinical Nutrition, 91*(5), 1461S-1467S. https://doi.org/10.3945/ajcn.2010.28674F

Indiana University. (n.d.). Iron consumption can increase risk for heart disease, study shows. Retrieved from ScienceDaily website: https://www.sciencedaily.com/releases/ 2014/04/140423170903.htm

Jeong, S.-H., Kim, J.-S., Kim, H.-J., Choi, J.-Y., Koo, J.-W., Choi, K.-D., Park, J.-Y., Lee, S.-H., Choi, S.-Y., Oh, S.-Y., Yang, T.-H., Park, J.H., Jung, I., Ahn, S., & Kim, S. (2020). Prevention of benign paroxysmal positional vertigo with vit D supplementation: A randomized trial. *Neurology,* 10.1212/WNL.0000000000010343. https://doi.org/10.1212/ WNL.0000000000010343

Kerr, D.C.R., Zava, D.T., Piper, W.T., Saturn, S.R., Frei, B., & Gombart, A.F. (2015). Associations between vitamin D levels and depressive symptoms in healthy young adult women. *Psychiatry Research, 227*(1), 46–51. https://doi.org/10.1016/j.psychres.2015.02.016

Lents, N.H. (n.d.). The evolutionary quirk that made vitamin B12 part of our diet. Retrieved from Discover Magazine website: https://www.discovermagazine.com/ health/the-evolutionary-quirk-that-made-vitamin-b12-part-of-our-diet

Linus Pauling biography. (2014, May 9). Retrieved from Linus Pauling Institute website: https://lpi.oregonstate.edu/about/linus-pauling-biography

Linus Pauling Institute. (n.d.). Retrieved from Linus Pauling Institute website: https://lpi. oregonstate.edu/

Maghbooli, Z., Sahraian, M.A., Ebrahimi, M., Pazoki, M., Kafan, S., Tabriz, H.M., Hadadi, A., Montazeri, M., Nasiri, M., Shirvani, A., & Holick, M.F. (2020). Vitamin D sufficiency, a serum 25-hydroxyvitamin D at least 30 ng/mL reduced risk for adverse clinical outcomes in patients with COVID-19 infection. *PLOS ONE, 15*(9), e0239799. https://doi.org/10.1371/ journal.pone.0239799

Martini, F., Ober, W., Nath, J., Bartholomew, E., & Petti, K. (2018). *Visual anatomy & physiology* (3rd edition). NY, NY: Pearson.

Mursu, J. (2011). Dietary supplements and mortality rate in older women: The Iowa Women's Health Study. *Archives of Internal Medicine, 171*(18), 1625. https://doi.org/10.1001/ archinternmed.2011.445

National Archives at Atlanta. (n.d.). Retrieved from https://www.archives.gov/atlanta/ exhibits/item470-full.html

Office of Dietary Supplements (ODS). (n.d.). Retrieved from https://ods.od.nih.gov/index.aspx

Office on Women's Health. (2016, August 16). Retrieved from Womenshealth.gov website: https://www.womenshealth.gov/office-womens-health

Offit, P.A. (2013). *Do you believe in magic? The sense and nonsense of alternative medicine* (First edition). New York: Harper.

Offit, P.A. (2014). *Do you believe in magic?: Vitamins, supplements, and all things natural: A look behind the curtain.* HarperCollins.

Price, C. (2017, August 14). The age of scurvy. Retrieved from Science History Institute website: https://www.sciencehistory.org/distillations/the-age-of-scurvy

Raffensperger, L. (2013, July 23). How adding iodine to salt boosted americans' iq.

Ran, L., Zhao, W., Wang, J., Wang, H., Zhao, Y., Tseng, Y., & Bu, H. (2018). Extra dose of vitamin C based on a daily supplementation shortens the common cold: A meta-analysis of 9 randomized controlled trials. *BioMed Research International, 2018,* 1837634. https://doi. org/10.1155/2018/1837634

Reference standards | USP. (n.d.). Retrieved from https://www.usp.org/reference-standards

Roguin Maor, N., Alperin, M., Shturman, E., Khairaldeen, H., Friedman, M., Karkabi,

K., & Milman, U. (2017). Effect of magnesium oxide supplementation on nocturnal leg cramps: a randomized clinical trial. *JAMA Internal Medicine, 177*(5), 617–623. https://doi.org/10.1001/jamainternmed.2016.9261

Sami, A., & Abrahamsen, B. (2019). The latest evidence from vitamin D intervention trials for skeletal and non-skeletal outcomes. *Calcified Tissue International.* https://doi.org/10.1007/s00223–019–00616-y

Singh, S., & Ernst, E. (2008). *Trick or treatment: The undeniable facts about alternative medicine* (1st American ed). New York: W.W. Norton.

Supakatisant, C., & Phupong, V. (2015). Oral magnesium for relief in pregnancy-induced leg cramps: A randomised controlled trial. *Maternal & Child Nutrition, 11*(2), 139–145. https://doi.org/10.1111/j.1740–8709.2012.00440.x

Tuskegee Study—Timeline—CDC—NCHHSTP. (2020, July 16). https://www.cdc.gov/timeline.htm

Wienecke, E., & Nolden, C. (2016). [Long-term HRV analysis shows stress reduction by magnesium intake]. *MMW Fortschritte der Medizin, 158*(Suppl 6), 12–16. https://doi.org/10.1007/s15006–016–9054–7

Chapter 8

Ahl, J. (n.d.). Bayer looking to expand Dicamba use to corn despite lawsuit, drift damage. Retrieved from https://www.harvestpublicmedia.org/post/bayer-looking-expand-dicamba-use-corn-despite-lawsuit-drift-damage

Aquifers and groundwater. (n.d.). Retrieved from https://www.usgs.gov/special-topic/water-science-school/science/aquifers-and-groundwater?qt-science_center_objects=0#qt-science_center_objects

Bayer completes Monsanto acquisition. (2018, June 8). Retrieved from Farm Progress website: https://www.farmprogress.com/business/bayer-completes-monsanto-acquisition

Biotechnology FAQs. (n.d.). Retrieved from https://www.usda.gov/topics/biotechnology/biotechnology-frequently-asked-questions-faqs

Brkić, D., Szakonyne-Pasics, I., Gašić, S., Teodorović, I., Rašković, B., Brkić, N., & Nešković, N. (2015). Subacute and subchronic toxicity of Avalon(*) mixture (bentazone+dicamba) to rats. *Environmental Toxicology and Pharmacology, 39*(3), 1057–1066. https://doi.org/10.1016/j.etap.2015.03.004

CDC. (2019, March 11). Antibiotic resistance and food are connected. Retrieved from Centers for Disease Control and Prevention website: https://www.cdc.gov/drugresistance/food.html

CDC. (2019, August 27). Four simple steps to food safety. Retrieved from Centers for Disease Control and Prevention website: https://www.cdc.gov/foodsafety/keep-food-safe.html

Cohen, P. (2020, June 24). Roundup maker to pay $10 billion to settle cancer suits. *The New York Times.* https://www.nytimes.com/2020/06/24/business/roundup-settlement-lawsuits.html

Cuppari, C., Manti, S., Salpietro, A., Dugo, G., Gitto, E., Arrigo, T., … Salpietro, C. (2015). Almond milk: A potential therapeutic weapon against cow's milk protein allergy. *Journal of Biological Regulators and Homeostatic Agents, 29*(2 Suppl 1), 8–12.

Dairy | Industries | WWF. (n.d.). Retrieved from World Wildlife Fund website: https://www.worldwildlife.org/industries/dairy

Domex Superfresh Growers. Retrieved from https://superfreshgrowers.com/about-us

Environmental Working Group. (n.d.). Retrieved from EWG website: https://www.ewg.org/about-us

Freydier, L., & Lundgren, J.G. (2016). Unintended effects of the herbicides 2,4-D and dicamba on lady beetles. *Ecotoxicology (London, England), 25*(6), 1270–1277. https://doi.org/10.1007/s10646–016–1680–4

GM crops can lift farmers out of poverty, study shows. (n.d.). Alliance for Science. Retrieved from https://allianceforscience.cornell.edu/blog/2020/08/gm-crops-can-lift-farmers-out-of-poverty-study-shows/

Heat treatments and pasteurization | MilkFacts.info. (n.d.). Retrieved from http://milkfacts. info/Milk%20Processing/Heat%20Treatments%20and%20Pasteurization.htm

How much water do cows drink. (n.d.). Retrieved from UNL Beef website: https://beef.unl. edu/amountwatercowsdrink

How much water is there on earth? (n.d.). Retrieved from https://www.usgs.gov/special-topic/water-science-school/science/how-much-water-there-earth?qt-science_center_objects=0#qt-science_center_objects

Jirillo, F., & Magrone, T. (2014). Anti-inflammatory and anti-allergic properties of donkey's and goat's milk. *Endocrine, Metabolic & Immune Disorders Drug Targets, 14*(1), 27–37. https://doi.org/10.2174/1871530314666140121143747

Michel, J. (n.d.). U.S. officials face growing pressure over dicamba herbicide use. Retrieved from https://phys.org/news/2018-09-pressure-dicamba-herbicide.html

Mills, P.J., Kania-Korwel, I., Fagan, J., McEvoy, L.K., Laughlin, G.A., & Barrett-Connor, E. (2017). Excretion of the herbicide glyphosate in older adults between 1993 and 2016. *JAMA, 318*(16), 1610–1611. https://doi.org/10.1001/jama.2017.11726

Olson-Sawyer, K. (2013, December 16). Meat's large water footprint: Why raising livestock and poultry for meat is so resource-intensive. Retrieved from Food Tank website: https:// foodtank.com/news/2013/12/why-meat-eats-resources/

Pärnänen, K., Karkman, A., Hultman, J., Lyra, C., Bengtsson-Palme, J., Larsson, D.G.J., ... Virta, M. (2018). Maternal gut and breast milk microbiota affect infant gut antibiotic resistome and mobile genetic elements. *Nature Communications, 9*(1), 3891. https://doi. org/10.1038/s41467-018-06393-w

Polyface Farms. (n.d.). Principles. Retrieved from http://www.polyfacefarms.com/ principles/

Shelburne Farms. (2019, May 13). Cultivating pathways to sustainability. Retrieved from Shelburne Farms website: https://shelburnefarms.org/cultivating-pathways-to-sustainability

Smith-Schoenwalder, C. (n.d.). What you should know about glyphosate, the pesticide in Roundup weed killer. Retrieved from US News & World Report website: https://www. usnews.com/news/national-news/articles/what-to-know-about-glyphosate-the-pesticide-in-roundup-weed-killer

Sustainable Agriculture | National Institute of Food and Agriculture. (n.d.). Retrieved from https://nifa.usda.gov/topic/sustainable-agriculture

Tarazona, J.V., Court-Marques, D., Tiramani, M., Reich, H., Pfeil, R., Istace, F., & Crivellente, F. (2017). Glyphosate toxicity and carcinogenicity: A review of the scientific basis of the European Union assessment and its differences with IARC. *Archives of Toxicology, 91*(8), 2723–2743. https://doi.org/10.1007/s00204-017-1962-5

USDA ERS—Irrigation & Water Use. (n.d.). Retrieved from https://www.ers.usda.gov/topics/ farm-practices-management/irrigation-water-use.aspx

USDA Organic Integrity Database. (n.d.). Retrieved from https://organic.ams.usda.gov/ integrity/

Valtin, H., & (With the Technical Assistance of Sheila A. Gorman). (2002). "Drink at least eight glasses of water a day." Really? Is there scientific evidence for "8 × 8"? *American Journal of Physiology-Regulatory, Integrative and Comparative Physiology, 283*(5), R993–R1004. https://doi.org/10.1152/ajpregu.00365.2002

Water availability and distribution for livestock. (n.d.). Retrieved from https://web.archive. org/web/20151117070950/http://www.noble.org/ag/livestock/waterconcerns/

Water scarcity: Economic implications | Water Resource | Water Economy. (n.d.). Retrieved from https://web.archive.org/web/20151201220321/http://growingblue.com/implications-of-growth/economic-implications/

What is sustainable agriculture? (n.d.). Retrieved from Union of Concerned Scientists website: https://www.ucsusa.org/resources/what-sustainable-agriculture

Woman dies after water-drinking contest. (2007, January 14). Retrieved November 11, 2019, from Msnbc.com website: http://www.nbcnews.com/id/16614865/ns/us_news-life/t/ woman-dies-after-water-drinking-contest/

Chapter 9

Adler, D.G. (n.d.). The grim origins of "gluten-free" | DiscoverMagazine.com. Retrieved from Discover Magazine website: http://discovermagazine.com/2019/may/the-grim-origins-of-gluten-free

Barna, M. (n.d.). The science behind fasting diets. Discover Magazine. Retrieved from https://www.discovermagazine.com/health/fasting-may-be-more-than-a-fad-diet

Bloomfield, H.E., Koeller, E., Greer, N., MacDonald, R., Kane, R., & Wilt, T.J. (2016). Effects on health outcomes of a Mediterranean Diet with no restriction on fat intake: A systematic review and meta-analysis. *Annals of Internal Medicine, 165*(7), 491. https://doi.org/10.7326/M16–0361

Burgess, N.S. (1991). Effect of a very-low-calorie diet on body composition and resting metabolic rate in obese men and women. *Journal of the American Dietetic Association, 91*(4), 430–434.

Chin, S.O., Keum, C., Woo, J., Park, J., Choi, H.J., Woo, J., & Rhee, S.Y. (2016). Successful weight reduction and maintenance by using a smartphone application in those with overweight and obesity. *Scientific Reports, 6*(1), 34563. https://doi.org/10.1038/srep34563

CNN, S.L. (n.d.). Half of America will be obese within 10 years, study says, unless we work together. Retrieved from CNN website: https://www.cnn.com/2019/12/18/health/american-obesity-trends-wellness/index.html

Corella, D., Carrasco, P., Sorlí, J. V., Estruch, R., Rico-Sanz, J., Martínez-González, M.Á., … Ordovás, J.M. (2013). Mediterranean Diet reduces the adverse effect of the TCF7L2-rs7903146 polymorphism on cardiovascular risk factors and stroke incidence: A randomized controlled trial in a high-cardiovascular-risk population. *Diabetes Care.* https://doi.org/10.2337/dc13–0955

Editor. (2019, January 15). Diabetic retinopathy usually only affects people who have had diabetes (diagnosed or undiagnosed) for a significant number of years. Retrieved from Diabetes website: https://www.diabetes.co.uk/diabetes-complications/diabetic-retinopathy.html

"Freshman 15" weight gain is a myth: Study. (2011, November 1). *Reuters.* Retrieved from https://www.reuters.com/article/us-college-weight-idUSTRE7A055O20111101

Ge, L., Sadeghirad, B., Ball, G.D.C., da Costa, B.R., Hitchcock, C.L., Svendrovski, A., Kiflen, R., Quadri, K., Kwon, H.Y., Karamouzian, M., Adams-Webber, T., Ahmed, W., Damanhoury, S., Zeraatkar, D., Nikolakopoulou, A., Tsuyuki, R.T., Tian, J., Yang, K., Guyatt, G.H., & Johnston, B.C. (2020). Comparison of dietary macronutrient patterns of 14 popular named dietary programmes for weight and cardiovascular risk factor reduction in adults: Systematic review and network meta-analysis of randomised trials. *BMJ*, m696. https://doi.org/10.1136/bmj.m696

Ghayur, M.N., & Gilani, A.H. (2005). Ginger lowers blood pressure through blockade of voltage-dependent calcium channels. *Journal of Cardiovascular Pharmacology, 45*(1), 74–80. https://doi.org/10.1097/00005344–200501000–00013

Grapefruit Diet—Weird Al. (n.d.). Retrieved from https://www.youtube.com/watch?v=zhfLfJCqrqI

Grapefruit Diets. (n.d.). Retrieved from https://web.archive.org/web/20090409065141/http://yourtotalhealth.ivillage.com/diet-fitness/grapefruit.html

Gudzune, K.A., Doshi, R.S., Mehta, A.K., Chaudhry, Z.W., Jacobs, D.K., Vakil, R.M., … Clark, J.M. (2015). Efficacy of commercial weight loss programs: An updated systematic review. *Annals of Internal Medicine, 162*(7), 501–512. https://doi.org/10.7326/M14–2238

Hermansen, K. (2000). Diet, blood pressure and hypertension. *The British Journal of Nutrition, 83 Suppl 1*, S113–119. https://doi.org/10.1017/s0007114500001045

How the Nutrisystem diet works | Top weight loss program. (n.d.). Retrieved from https://www.nutrisystem.com/jsps_hmr/how_it_works/index.jsp

Karmali, K.N., Lloyd-Jones, D.M., Berendsen, M.A., Goff, D.C., Sanghavi, D.M., Brown, N.C., … Huffman, M.D. (2016). Drugs for primary prevention of atherosclerotic cardiovascular disease: An overview of systematic reviews. *JAMA Cardiology, 1*(3), 341–349. https://doi.org/10.1001/jamacardio.2016.0218

Kertes, P.J., & Johnson, T.M. (Eds.). (2007). *Evidence-based eye care*. Philadelphia, PA: Lippincott Williams & Wilkins.

Kim, H., Patel, K.G., Orosz, E., Kothari, N., Demyen, M.F., Pyrsopoulos, N., & Ahlawat, S.K. (2016). Time trends in the prevalence of Celiac Disease and gluten-free diet in the U.S. population: Results from the National Health and Nutrition Examination Surveys 2009–2014. *JAMA Internal Medicine*, 176(11), 1716. https://doi.org/10.1001/jamainternmed.2016.5254

Koenig, D. (n.d.). Quarantine weight gain not a joking matter. WebMD. Retrieved from https://www.webmd.com/lung/news/20200521/quarantine-weight-gain-not-a-joking-matter

Maghbooli, M., Golipour, F., Moghimi Esfandabadi, A., & Yousefi, M. (2014). Comparison between the efficacy of ginger and sumatriptan in the ablative treatment of the common migraine: *Phytotherapy Research*, 28(3), 412–415. https://doi.org/10.1002/ptr.4996

Markey, C. (n.d.). Six myths about the freshman 15. Retrieved from US News & World Report website: https://health.usnews.com/health-news/blogs/eat-run/articles/2017-08-25/6-myths-about-the-freshman-15

Martínez-Lapiscina, E.H., Clavero, P., Toledo, E., Estruch, R., Salas-Salvadó, J., San Julián, B., … Martinez-Gonzalez, M. Á. (2013). Mediterranean diet improves cognition: The PREDIMED-NAVARRA randomised trial. *Journal of Neurology, Neurosurgery, and Psychiatry*, 84(12), 1318–1325. https://doi.org/10.1136/jnnp-2012-304792

Martins, L.B., Rodrigues, A.M. dos S., Rodrigues, D.F., dos Santos, L.C., Teixeira, A.L., & Ferreira, A.V.M. (2019). Double-blind placebo-controlled randomized clinical trial of ginger (*Zingiber officinale Rosc.*) addition in migraine acute treatment. *Cephalalgia*, 39(1), 68–76. https://doi.org/10.1177/0333102418776016

Mihalopoulos, N.L., Auinger, P., & Klein, J.D. (2008). The freshman 15: Is it real? *Journal of American College Health: J of ACH*, 56(5), 531–533. https://doi.org/10.3200/JACH.56.5.531–534

Müller, M.J., Enderle, J., & Bosy-Westphal, A. (2016). Changes in energy expenditure with weight gain and weight loss in humans. *Current Obesity Reports*, 5(4), 413–423. https://doi.org/10.1007/s13679-016-0237-4

Müller, M.J., Enderle, J., Pourhassan, M., Braun, W., Eggeling, B., Lagerpusch, M., … Bosy-Westphal, A. (2015). Metabolic adaptation to caloric restriction and subsequent refeeding: The Minnesota Starvation Experiment revisited. *The American Journal of Clinical Nutrition*, 102(4), 807–819. https://doi.org/10.3945/ajcn.115.109173

~~Noom Inc. (n.d.). Noom Inc. Retrieved from https://www.noom.com~~

Nordqvist, C. (2017). Nine most popular diets rated by experts 2017. *Medical News Today*.

Patel, M.L., Hopkins, C.M., Brooks, T.L., & Bennett, G.G. (2019). Comparing self-monitoring strategies for weight loss in a smartphone app: Randomized controlled trial. *JMIR MHealth and UHealth*, 7(2), e12209. https://doi.org/10.2196/12209

Pearl, R.L. (2020). Weight stigma and the "quarantine-15." *Obesity*, 28(7), 1180–1181. https://doi.org/10.1002/oby.22850

Rietsema, S., Eelderink, C., Joustra, M.L., van Vliet, I.M.Y., van Londen, M., Corpeleijn, E., … Bakker, S.J.L. (2019). Effect of high compared with low dairy intake on blood pressure in overweight middle-aged adults: Results of a randomized crossover intervention study. *The American Journal of Clinical Nutrition*, 110(2), 340–348. https://doi.org/10.1093/ajcn/nqz116

Sacks, F.M., Svetkey, L.P., Vollmer, W.M., Appel, L.J., Bray, G.A., Harsha, D., … DASH-Sodium Collaborative Research Group. (2001). Effects on blood pressure of reduced dietary sodium and the Dietary Approaches to Stop Hypertension (DASH) diet. DASH-Sodium Collaborative Research Group. *The New England Journal of Medicine*, 344(1), 3–10. https://doi.org/10.1056/NEJM200101043440101

Sala-Vila, A., Díaz-López, A., Valls-Pedret, C., Cofán, M., García-Layana, A., Lamuela-Raventós, R.-M., … Prevención con Dieta Mediterránea (PREDIMED) Investigators. (2016). Dietary marine ω-3 fatty acids and incident sight-threatening retinopathy in middle-aged and older individuals with type 2 diabetes: Prospective investigation from the PREDIMED trial. *JAMA Ophthalmology*, 134(10), 1142–1149. https://doi.org/10.1001/jamaophthalmol.2016.2906

Shannon, O.M., Stephan, B.C.M., Granic, A., Lentjes, M., Hayat, S., Mulligan, A., … Siervo, M. (2019). Mediterranean diet adherence and cognitive function in older UK adults: The

European Prospective Investigation into Cancer and Nutrition-Norfolk (EPIC-Norfolk) Study. *The American Journal of Clinical Nutrition, 110*(4), 938–948. https://doi.org/10.1093/ajcn/nqz114

Sutton, E.F., Beyl, R., Early, K.S., Cefalu, W.T., Ravussin, E., & Peterson, C.M. (2018). Early time-restricted feeding improves insulin sensitivity, blood pressure, and oxidative stress even without weight loss in men with prediabetes. *Cell Metabolism, 27*(6), 1212–1221.e3. https://doi.org/10.1016/j.cmet.2018.04.010

Syage, J.A., Kelly, C.P., Dickason, M.A., Ramirez, A.C., Leon, F., Dominguez, R., & Sealey-Voyksner, J.A. (2018). Determination of gluten consumption in Celiac Disease patients on a gluten-free diet. *The American Journal of Clinical Nutrition, 107*(2), 201–207. https://doi.org/10.1093/ajcn/nqx049

Taylor, K.B., & Anthony, L.E. (1983). *Clinical nutrition.* New York: McGraw-Hill.

Templeman, I., Gonzalez, J.T., Thompson, D., & Betts, J.A. (2019). The role of intermittent fasting and meal timing in weight management and metabolic health. *Proceedings of the Nutrition Society*, 1–12. https://doi.org/10.1017/S0029665119000636

Weight Loss Programs & Plans That Work | Jenny Craig. (n.d.). Retrieved from https://www.jennycraig.com/how-it-works

Williams, W.F. (2013). *Encyclopedia of pseudoscience: From alien abductions to zone therapy.* Hoboken: Taylor and Francis.

Zagorsky, J.L., & Smith, P.K. (2011). The freshman 15: A critical time for obesity intervention or media myth? *Social Science Quarterly, 92*(5), 1389–1407. https://doi.org/10.1111/j.1540-6237.2011.00823.x

Chapter 10

Abernethy, A. (2019). FDA is committed to sound, science-based policy on CBD. *FDA.* Retrieved from http://www.fda.gov/news-events/fda-voices-perspectives-fda-leadership-and-experts/fda-committed-sound-science-based-policy-cbd

Aizawa, N., Fujimori, Y., Kobayashi, J., Nakanishi, O., Hirasawa, H., Kume, H., Homma, Y., & Igawa, Y. (2018). KPR-2579, a novel TRPM8 antagonist, inhibits acetic acid-induced bladder afferent hyperactivity in rats. *Neurourology and Urodynamics, 37*(5), 1633–1640. https://doi.org/10.1002/nau.23532

Andreux, P.A., Blanco-Bose, W., Ryu, D., Burdet, F., Ibberson, M., Aebischer, P., ... Rinsch, C. (2019). The mitophagy activator urolithin A is safe and induces a molecular signature of improved mitochondrial and cellular health in humans. *Nature Metabolism, 1*(6), 595–603. https://doi.org/10.1038/s42255-019-0073-4

Arnett, D.K., Blumenthal, R.S., Albert, M.A., Buroker, A.B., Himmelfarb, C.D., Goldberger, Z.D., ... Ziaeian, B. (2019). A report of the American College of Cardiology/American Heart Association Task Force on Clinical Practice Guidelines. 17.

Aviram, M., & Dornfeld, L. (2001). Pomegranate juice consumption inhibits serum angiotensin converting enzyme activity and reduces systolic blood pressure. *Atherosclerosis, 158*(1), 195–198. https://doi.org/10.1016/S0021-9150(01)00412-9

Baddeley, B., Sornalingam, S., & Cooper, M. (2016). Sitting is the new smoking: Where do we stand? *The British Journal of General Practice, 66*(646), 258. https://doi.org/10.3399/bjgp16X685009

Bailey, B.W., Bartholomew, C.L., Summerhays, C., Deru, L., Compton, S., Tucker, L.A., LeCheminant, J.D., & Hicks, J. (2019). The impact of step recommendations on body composition and physical activity patterns in college freshman women: A randomized trial. *Journal of Obesity, 2019*, 1–8. https://doi.org/10.1155/2019/4036825

Barić, H., Đorđević, V., Cerovečki, I., & Trkulja, V. (2018). Complementary and alternative medicine treatments for Generalized Anxiety Disorder: Systematic review and meta-analysis of randomized controlled trials. *Advances in Therapy, 35*(3), 261–288. https://doi.org/10.1007/s12325-018-0680-6

Blackburn, L., Achor, S., Allen, B., Bauchmire, N., Dunnington, D., Klisovic, R., ... Chipps, E. (2017). The effect of aromatherapy on insomnia and other common symptoms among patients with Acute Leukemia. *Oncology Nursing Forum, 44*(4), E185–E193. https://doi.org/10.1188/17.ONF.E185-E193

Boggs, D.L., Nguyen, J.D., Morgenson, D., Taffe, M.A., & Ranganathan, M. (2018). Clinical and preclinical evidence for functional interactions of Cannabidiol and Δ 9 -Tetrahydrocannabinol. *Neuropsychopharmacology, 43*(1), 142–154. https://doi.org/10.1038/npp.2017.209

Caputo, L., Reguilon, M.D., Miñarro, J., De Feo, V., & Rodriguez-Arias, M. (2018). *Lavandula angustifolia* essential oil and linalool counteract social aversion induced by social defeat. *Molecules (Basel, Switzerland), 23*(10). https://doi.org/10.3390/molecules23102694

Carrigan, M.A., Uryasev, O., Frye, C.B., Eckman, B.L., Myers, C.R., Hurley, T.D., & Benner, S.A. (2015). Hominids adapted to metabolize ethanol long before human-directed fermentation. *Proceedings of the National Academy of Sciences, 112*(2), 458–463. https://doi.org/10.1073/pnas.1404167111

Cederbaum, A.I. (2012). Alcohol metabolism. *Clinics in Liver Disease, 16*(4), 667–685. https://doi.org/10.1016/j.cld.2012.08.002

Coffee consumption and health: Umbrella review of meta-analyses of multiple health outcomes. (2018). *BMJ, 360.* https://doi.org/10.1136/bmj.k194

d'Unienville, N.M.A., Hill, A.M., Coates, A.M., Yandell, C., Nelson, M.J., & Buckley, J.D. (2019). Effects of almond, dried grape and dried cranberry consumption on endurance exercise performance, recovery and psychomotor speed: Protocol of a randomised controlled trial. *BMJ Open Sport & Exercise Medicine, 5*(1), e000560. https://doi.org/10.1136/bmjsem-2019-000560

Erickson, M.L., Jenkins, N.T., & McCully, K.K. (2017). Exercise after you eat: Hitting the postprandial glucose target. *Frontiers in Endocrinology, 8.* https://doi.org/10.3389/fendo.2017.00228

Ernst, E., & Pittler, M.H. (2000). Efficacy of ginger for nausea and vomiting: A systematic review of randomized clinical trials. *BJA: British Journal of Anaesthesia, 84*(3), 367–371. https://doi.org/10.1093/oxfordjournals.bja.a013442

Fan, J., & Dowell, V. (n.d.). Move it and lose it: Every "brisk" minute counts. University of Utah News. Retrieved from https://archive.unews.utah.edu/news_releases/move-it-and-lose-it-every-brisk-minute-counts/

Final Recommendation Statement: Low-Dose aspirin use for the prevention of morbidity and mortality from preeclampsia: Preventive Medication—US Preventive Services Task Force. (n.d.). Retrieved from https://www.uspreventiveservicestaskforce.org/Page/Document/RecommendationStatementFinal/low-dose-aspirin-use-for-the-prevention-of-morbidity-and-mortality-from-preeclampsia-preventive-medication

Franco, L., Blanck, T.J.J., Dugan, K., Kline, R., Shanmugam, G., Galotti, A., ... Wajda, M. (2016). Both lavender fleur oil and unscented oil aromatherapy reduce preoperative anxiety in breast surgery patients: A randomized trial. *Journal of Clinical Anesthesia, 33,* 243–249. https://doi.org/10.1016/j.jclinane.2016.02.032

Futterman, M. (2016, July 11). A new way to prevent muscle cramps. *WSJ.* https://www.wsj.com/articles/a-new-way-to-prevent-muscle-cramps-1468256588

Gray, S.L., Anderson, M.L., Dublin, S., Hanlon, J.T., Hubbard, R., Walker, R., ... Larson, E.B. (2015). Cumulative use of strong anticholinergics and incident dementia: A prospective cohort study. *JAMA Internal Medicine, 175*(3), 401–407. https://doi.org/10.1001/jamainternmed.2014.7663

Hafez, E.M., Hamad, M.A., Fouad, M., & Abdel-Lateff, A. (2017). Auto-brewery Syndrome: Ethanol pseudo-toxicity in diabetic and hepatic patients. *Human & Experimental Toxicology, 36*(5), 445–450. https://doi.org/10.1177/0960327116661400

Hojman, P., Gehl, J., Christensen, J.F., & Pedersen, B.K. (2018). Molecular mechanisms linking exercise to cancer prevention and treatment. *Cell Metabolism, 27*(1), 10–21. https://doi.org/10.1016/j.cmet.2017.09.015

Holmstrup, M.E., Fairchild, T.J., Keslacy, S., Weinstock, R.S., & Kanaley, J.A. (2013). Satiety, but not total PYY, is increased with continuous and intermittent exercise. *Obesity, 21*(10), 2014–2020. https://doi.org/10.1002/oby.20335

Irish, L.A., Kline, C.E., Gunn, H.E., Buysse, D.J., & Hall, M.H. (2015). The role of sleep hygiene in promoting public health: A review of empirical evidence. *Sleep Medicine Reviews, 22*, 23–36. https://doi.org/10.1016/j.smrv.2014.10.001

Jansson-Nettelbladt, E., Meurling, S., Petrini, B., & Sjölin, J. (2006). Endogenous ethanol fermentation in a child with short bowel syndrome. *Acta Paediatrica, 95*(4), 502–504. https://doi.org/10.1080/08035250500501625

Knufinke, M., Nieuwenhuys, A., Geurts, S.A.E., Coenen, A.M.L., & Kompier, M.A.J. (2018). Self-reported sleep quantity, quality and sleep hygiene in elite athletes. *Journal of Sleep Research, 27*(1), 78–85. https://doi.org/10.1111/jsr.12509

Lambert, J. (2019, November 5). Running just once a week may help you outpace an early death. Retrieved from Science News website: https://www.sciencenews.org/article/running-just-once-week-may-help-you-avoid-early-death

Lopresti, A.L., Smith, S.J., Malvi, H., & Kodgule, R. (2019). An investigation into the stress-relieving and pharmacological actions of an ashwagandha (*Withania somnifera*) extract: A randomized, double-blind, placebo-controlled study. *Medicine, 98*(37), e17186. https://doi.org/10.1097/MD.0000000000017186

Malcolm, B.J., & Tallian, K. (2017). Essential oil of lavender in anxiety disorders: Ready for prime time? *The Mental Health Clinician, 7*(4), 147–155. https://doi.org/10.9740/mhc.2017.07.147

Nishimura, M., Suzuki, M., Takahashi, R., Yamaguchi, S., Tsubaki, K., Fujita, T., Nishihira, J., & Nakamura, K. (2019). Daily ingestion of eggplant powder improves blood pressure and psychological state in stressed individuals: A randomized placebo-controlled study. *Nutrients, 11*(11), 2797. https://doi.org/10.3390/nu11112797

Painter, K., Cordell, B., & Sticco, K.L. (2019). Auto-brewery Syndrome (Gut Fermentation). In *StatPearls*. Retrieved from http://www.ncbi.nlm.nih.gov/books/NBK513346/

Pedisic, Z., Shrestha, N., Kovalchik, S., Stamatakis, E., Liangruenrom, N., Grgic, J., … Oja, P. (2019). Is running associated with a lower risk of all-cause, cardiovascular and cancer mortality, and is the more the better? A systematic review and meta-analysis. *British Journal of Sports Medicine*. https://doi.org/10.1136/bjsports-2018-100493

Physical activity reduces stress | Anxiety and Depression Association of America, ADAA. (n.d.). Retrieved from https://adaa.org/understanding-anxiety/related-illnesses/other-related-conditions/stress/physical-activity-reduces-st

Rambaldi, A., Jacobs, B.P., & Gluud, C. (2007). Milk thistle for alcoholic and/or hepatitis B or C virus liver diseases. *Cochrane Database of Systematic Reviews* (4). https://doi.org/10.1002/14651858.CD003620.pub3

Rasines-Perea, Z., & Teissedre, P.-L. (2017). Grape polyphenols' effects in human cardiovascular diseases and diabetes. *Molecules (Basel, Switzerland), 22*(1). https://doi.org/10.3390/molecules22010068

Resveratrol in prostate diseases—A short review. (2013). *Central European Journal of Urology*. https://doi.org/10.5173/ceju.2013.02.art8

Rôas, Y.A. dos S., Fernandes, C.A.M., & Reis, E.J.B. dos. (2019). Effect of exercise on body composition, lipid and glucose and blood pressure in women with chronic degenerative diseases. *J. Health Sci. (Londrina)*. Retrieved from http://revista.pgsskroton.com.br/index.php/JHealthSci/article/view/5486/4528

Sahebkar, A., Ferri, C., Giorgini, P., Bo, S., Nachtigal, P., & Grassi, D. (2017). Effects of pomegranate juice on blood pressure: A systematic review and meta-analysis of randomized controlled trials. *Pharmacological Research, 115*, 149–161. https://doi.org/10.1016/j.phrs.2016.11.018

Salehi, B., Mishra, A.P., Nigam, M., Sener, B., Kilic, M., Sharifi-Rad, M., … Sharifi-Rad, J. (2018). Resveratrol: A double-edged sword in health benefits. *Biomedicines, 6*(3). https://doi.org/10.3390/biomedicines6030091

Schmidt, M. (n.d.). Why walking might be one of the best exercises for health. Discover Magazine. Retrieved from https://www.discovermagazine.com/health/why-walking-might-be-one-of-the-best-exercises-for-health

Schmitz, K.H., Campbell, A.M., Stuiver, M.M., Pinto, B.M., Schwartz, A.L., Morris, G.S., … Matthews, C.E. (2019). Exercise is medicine in oncology: Engaging clinicians to help patients move through cancer. *CA: A Cancer Journal for Clinicians, 69*(6), 468–484. https://doi.org/10.3322/caac.21579

Schnohr, P., O'Keefe, J.H., Marott, J.L., Lange, P., & Jensen, G.B. (2015). Dose of jogging and long-term mortality: The Copenhagen City heart study. *Journal of the American College of Cardiology, 65*(5), 411–419. https://doi.org/10.1016/j.jacc.2014.11.023

Schwarzinger, M., Pollock, B.G., Hasan, O.S.M., Dufouil, C., Rehm, J., Baillot, S., ... Luchini, S. (2018). Contribution of alcohol use disorders to the burden of dementia in France 2008–13: a nationwide retrospective cohort study. *The Lancet Public Health, 3*(3), e124–e132. https://doi.org/10.1016/S2468-2667(18)30022-7

This gut bacteria makes people drunk without drinking—and causes liver disease. (2019, September 19). Retrieved from D-brief website: http://blogs.discovermagazine.com/d-brief/2019/09/19/auto-brewery-syndrome-gut-bacteria-liver-disease/

Tóth, B., Lantos, T., Hegyi, P., Viola, R., Vasas, A., Benkő, R., ... Csupor, D. (2018). Ginger (*Zingiber officinale*): An alternative for the prevention of postoperative nausea and vomiting. A meta-analysis. *Phytomedicine, 50*, 8–18. https://doi.org/10.1016/j.phymed.2018.09.007

Ventura-Cots, M., Watts, A.E., Cruz-Lemini, M., Shah, N.D., Ndugga, N., McCann, P., ... Bataller, R. (2019). Colder weather and fewer sunlight hours increase alcohol consumption and alcoholic cirrhosis worldwide. *Hepatology, 69*(5), 1916–1930. https://doi.org/10.1002/hep.30315

Welch, B.T., Coelho Prabhu, N., Walkoff, L., & Trenkner, S.W. (2016). Auto-brewery Syndrome in the setting of long-standing Crohn's Disease: A case report and review of the literature. *Journal of Crohn's and Colitis, 10*(12), 1448–1450. https://doi.org/10.1093/ecco-jcc/jjw098

Why Do We Sleep, Anyway? | Healthy Sleep. (n.d.). Retrieved from http://healthysleep.med.harvard.edu/healthy/matters/benefits-of-sleep/why-do-we-sleep

Williamson, A., & Feyer, A. (2000). Moderate sleep deprivation produces impairments in cognitive and motor performance equivalent to legally prescribed levels of alcohol intoxication. *Occupational and Environmental Medicine, 57*(10), 649–655. https://doi.org/10.1136/oem.57.10.649

World Health Organization model list of essential medicines: 21st list 2019. (n.d.). Retrieved from https://apps.who.int/iris/handle/10665/325771

Yamaguchi, S., Matsumoto, K., Koyama, M., Tian, S., Watanabe, M., Takahashi, A., Miyatake, K., & Nakamura, K. (2019). Antihypertensive effects of orally administered eggplant (*Solanum melongena*) rich in acetylcholine on spontaneously hypertensive rats. *Food Chemistry, 276*, 376–382. https://doi.org/10.1016/j.foodchem.2018.10.017

Zaccardi, F., Davies, M.J., Khunti, K., & Yates, T. (2019). Comparative relevance of physical fitness and adiposity on life expectancy. *Mayo Clinic Proceedings, 94*(6), 985–994. https://doi.org/10.1016/j.mayocp.2018.10.029

Index

Numbers in **bold italics** indicate pages with illustrations